Fundamentals of
Pharmaceutics and Dispensing Pharmacy

(Theory with Practical Applications)

Fundamentals of Pharmaceutics and Dispensing Pharmacy

(Theory with Practical Applications)

Dr. Honey Goel

An Alumnus of Department of Pharmaceutical Sciences and Drug Research,
Punjabi University, Patiala

Vinni Kalra

Research Scholar,
Department of Pharmaceutical Sciences and Drug Research,
Punjabi University, Patiala.

Dr. Ashok Kumar Tiwary

An Alumnus of Department of Pharmaceutical Sciences, BIT, Mesra,
Ranchi Department of Pharmaceutical Sciences and Drug Research of Punjabi
University

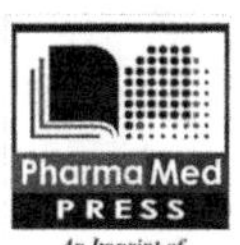

PharmaMed Press

An imprint of BSP Books pvt. Ltd
4-4-309/316, Giriraj Lane,
Sultan Bazar, Hyderabad - 500 095.

Fundamentals of Pharmaceutics & Dispensing Pharmacy
(Theory with practical applications)
by Dr. Honey Goel, Vinni Kalra and Dr. Ashok Kumar Tiwary

© 2024, *by Publisher*

Disclaimer: The authors and the publishers have taken due care to provide the authentic, reliable and up to date information related to the subject. However, neither the authors nor the publisher shall be responsible for any liability for any damage caused as a result of use of this book. The respective user must check the accuracy from other sources too.

Published by:

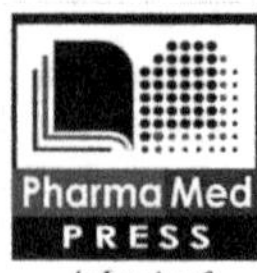

PharmaMed Press
An imprint of BSP Books Pvt. Ltd.
4-4-309/316, Giriraj Lane, Sultan Bazar, Hyderabad - 500 095.
Phone: 040-23445688; Fax: 91+40-23445611
e-mail: info@pharmamedpress.com
www.pharmamedpress.com/pharmamedpress.net

ISBN: 978-93-95039-78-9 (Hardback)

Preface

'Fundamentals of Pharmaceutics and Dispensing Pharmacy' is a new companion among vast literature created for undergraduate pharmacy students, teachers and colleagues working in the pharmacy profession. This book is intended to be used in conjunction with textbooks and reference books as an aid to provide practical application of dispensing pharmacy along with theoretical knowledge in order to help and understand the nitties and gritties of dispensing pharmacy.

This book has been written as a student guide to extemporaneous pharmaceutical compounding and dispensing. It has been designed to assist and cater the essential elements of an ideal pharmacy professional by understanding the key dosage forms and the challenges encountered within extemporaneous dispensing (including labeling and packaging). In addition, worked examples thoroughly tested in the laboratories have been included to allow the student to practice extemporaneous formulation exercises.

The present book is an attempt to provide essential information and awareness to a fresh entrant in B. Pharm. under graduate course (in compliance with PCI, Indian Pharmacopeia standards), required in dispensing pharmacy. This book will also be useful for preparing for the GPAT candidates, and to practicing pharmacists as a quick reference text.

- Authors

Contents

Unit 1

Basic Concepts of Dispensing

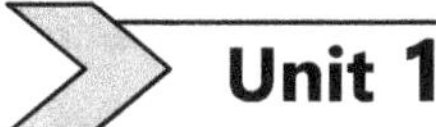 # Unit 1

Basic Concepts of Dispensing

General Introduction and Historical Background

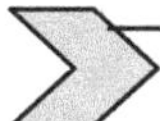 ### History of Pharmacy Profession in India

In ancient India the sources of drugs were of vegetable, animal and mineral origin. They were prepared empirically by few experienced persons. Knowledge of that medical system was usually kept secret within a family.

There were no scientific methods of standardization of drugs.

Muslim rule in India

The Indian system of medicine declined during the Muslim rule while the Arabic or the Unani-Tibbi system flourished.

British rule in India

The western or the so-called Allopathic system came into India with the British traders who later become the rulers. Under British rule this system got state patronage. At that time it was meant for the ruling race only. Later it descended to the people and become popular by the close of 19th Century.

Before 1940

Initially all the drugs were imported from Europe. Later some drugs of this system began to be manufactured in this country.

1901: Establishment of the Bengal Chemical and Pharmaceutical Works, Calcutta by Acharya P.C. Ray.

1903: A small factory at Parel (Bombay) by Prof. T.K. Gujjar.

1907: Alembic Chemical Works at Baroda by Prof. T.K. Gujjar.

Drugs were mostly exported in crude form and imported in finished form. During World War-I (1914 – 1920) the imports of drugs were cut-off. Imports of drugs were resumed after the War. In absence of any restrictions on quality of drugs imported, manufacturers abroad took advantage of the situation. The consequences were as follows:

(i) Foreign manufacturers dumped inferior quality medicines and adulterated drugs.

(ii) Markets were full of all sorts of useless and deleterious drugs which were sold by unqualified men.

Examples of maladies:

- Poisoning due to quinine.

- Putting of croton oil into eye instead of atropine solution.

- Selling of chalk powder tablets in place of quinine.

- Drug santonin was badly adulterated.

- Potent drugs like compounds of antimony and arsenic and preparations of digitalis were dispensed without any standard.

Few laws were promulgated, but they proved insufficient.

1878	Opium Act	Dealt with cultivation of poppy and the manufacture, transport, export, import and sale of opium.
1889	Indian Merchandise Act	Misbranding of goods in general
1894	Indian Tariff Act	Levy of customs duty on goods including foods, drinks, drugs, chemicals and medicines imported into India or exported there from.
1898	Sea Customs Act	Goods with 'false trade description' were prevented from importing under this act.
1860	Indian Penal Code	Some sections of IPC have mention of intentional adulterations as punishable offence.
1919	Poisons Act	Regulated the import, possession and sale of poisons.

Some state-level law had indirect references to drugs:

1884	Bengal Municipal Act	
1901	City of Bombay District Municipal Act	Concerned with food.
1909	Bengal Excise Act	
1911	Punjab Municipal Act	
1912	United Provinces (now Uttar Pradesh) Prevention of Adulteration Act	Refers to adulteration of foods and drugs.
1914	Pujab Excise Act	
1916	United Provinces Municipalities Act	Inspection of shops and seizure of adulterated substances.
1919	Bengal Food Adulteration Act	

Contd...

1919	Bihar and Orissa Prevention of Adulteration Act	
1919	Madras Prevention of Adulteration Act	Chiefly concerned with food adulteration
1922	Bihar and Orissa Municipal Act	
1922	Central Provinces Municipalities Act	
1925	Bombay Prevention of Adulteration Act	
1929	Punjab Pure Food Act	

The laws were too superficial and had indirect link to drugs.

Drug enquiry committee

Government of India on 11th August 1930, appointed a committee under the chairmanship of Late Col. R.N. Chopra to look into the problems of Pharmacy in India and recommend the measures to be taken. This committee published its report in 1931. It was reported that there was no recognized specialized profession of Pharmacy. A set of people known as compounders were filling the gap.

Just after the publication of the report Prof. Mahadeva Lal Schroff initiated pharmaceutical education at the university level in the Banaras Hindu University.

In 1935 United Province Pharmaceutical Association was established which later converted into Indian Pharmaceutical Association.

The Indian Journal of Pharmacy was started by Prof. M.L. Schroff in 1939. All India Pharmaceutical Congress Association was established in 1940. The Pharmaceutical Conference held its sessions at different places to publicize Pharmacy as a whole in India.

1937: Government of India brought 'Import of Drugs Bill'; later it was withdrawn.

1940: Govt. brought 'Drugs Bill' to regulate the import, manufacture, sale and distribution of drugs in British India. This Bill was finally adopted as 'Drugs Act of 1940'.

1941: The first Drugs Technical Advisory Board (D.T.A.B.) under this act was constituted.

Central Drugs Laboratory was established in Calcutta

1945:   'Drugs Rule under the Drugs Act of 1940' was established.

The Drugs Act has been modified from time to time and at present the provisions of the Act cover Cosmetics and Ayurvedic, Unani and Homeopathic medicines in some respects.

1945:   Government brought the Pharmacy Bill to standardize the Pharmacy Education in India.

1946:   The Indian Pharmacopoeial List was published under the chairmanship of late Col. R.N. Chopra. It contains lists of drugs in use in India at those times which were not included in British Pharmacopoeia.

1948:   Pharmacy Act 1948 was enacted on 04-03-1948 with the following preamble- "An Act to regulate the profession of pharmacy.

1948:   Indian Pharmacopoeial Committee was constituted under the chairmanship of late Dr. B.N. Ghosh.

1949:   Pharmacy Council of India (P.C.I.) was established under Pharmacy Act 1948.

1954:   Education Regulation came into force in some states, but many states lagged behind.

1954:   Drugs and Magic Remedies (Objectionable Advertisements) Act 1954 was passed to stop misleading advertisements (e.g. Cure all pills)

1955:   Medicinal and Toilet Preparations (Excise Duties) Act no. 16 of 1955 was introduced to enforce uniform collection of levy and duties of excise on medicinal and toilet preparation (alcohol products) in all states.

1955:   First Edition of Indian Pharmacopoeia was published.

1985:   Narcotic and Psychotropic Substances Act was enacted to protect society from the dangers of addictive drugs.

Government of India controls the price of drugs in India through Drugs Price Order changed from time to time.

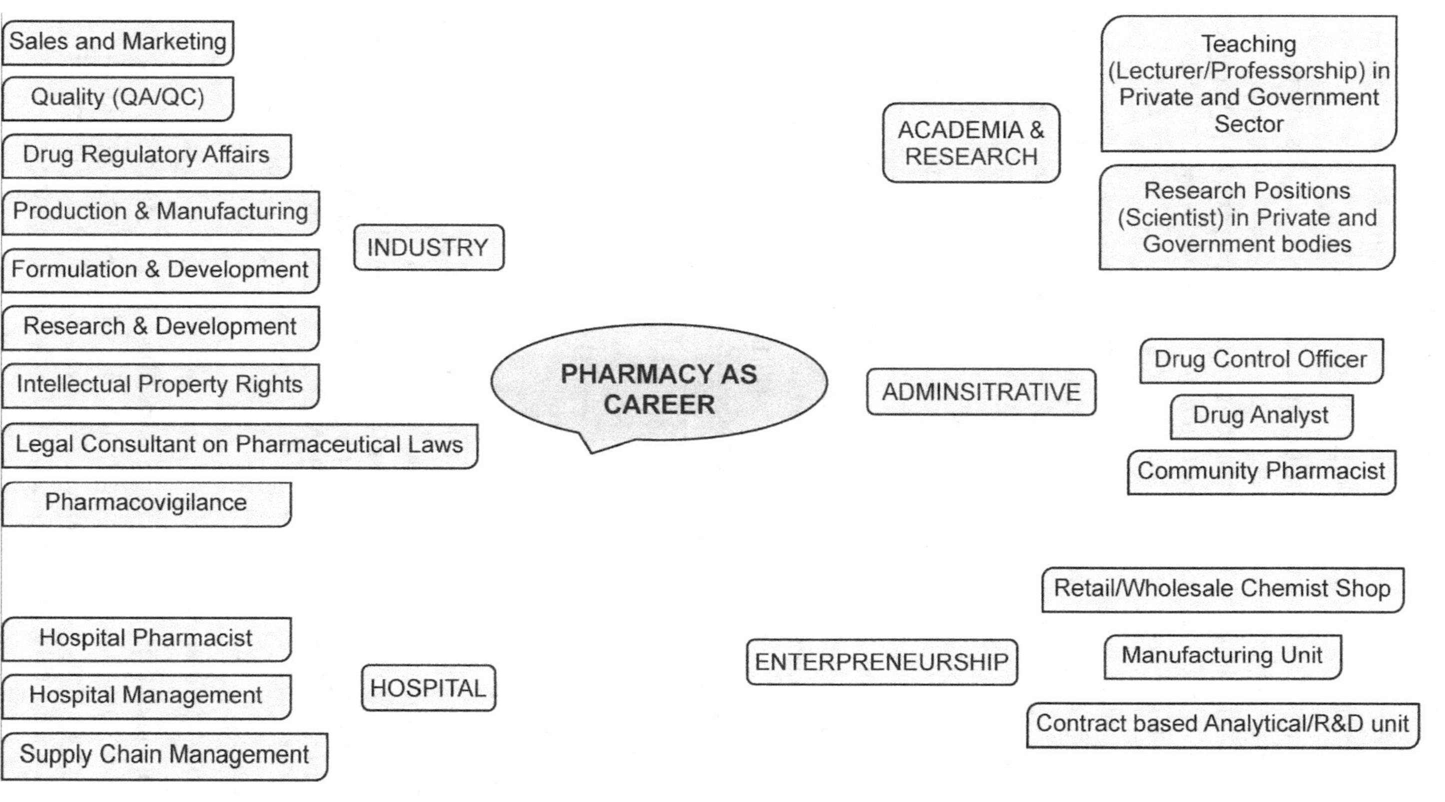

PHARMACY AS CAREER
INDUSTRY
Sales and Marketing
Quality (QA/QC)
Drug Regulatory Affairs
Production & Manufacturing
Formulation & Development
Research & Development
Intellectual Property Rights
Legal Consultant on Pharmaceutical Laws
Pharmacovigilance
HOSPITAL
Hospital Pharmacist
Hospital Management
Supply Chain Management
ACADEMIA & RESEARCH
Teaching (Lecturer/Professorship) in Private and Government Sector
Research Positions (Scientist) in Private and Government bodies
ADMINSITRATIVE
Drug Control Officer
Drug Analyst
Community Pharmacist
ENTERPRENEURSHIP
Retail/Wholesale Chemist Shop
Manufacturing Unit
Contract based Analytical/R&D unit

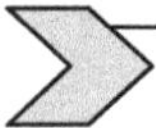 **Pharmacopoeia / Formularies / Compendia**

The term *"pharmacopoeia"* is derived from the Greek language *'pharmacon'* meaning 'drug' and *'poieo'* means 'to make'.

Literally, it is the written compilation or list of standards for drugs/medicinal substances/crude drugs or other related substances with approval from the drug regulatory authorities of the respective government in the country and termed as *pharmacopoeia* and *formularies* - collectively these standard text/reference books are known as the *drug compendia.*

Such drug compendia comprise a list of drugs and other related substances regarding their source, descriptions, standards, tests, formulae for concoting the same, action and uses, doses, storage conditions etc. These reference text books are revised and amended from time to time so as to incorporate the latest information regarding drugs or substances of therapeutic activity. For the preparation of these standard reference materials, expert reviews and opinions are taken from diverse segment of medical practitioners, teachers, pharmaceutical manufacturers and other stakeholders associated with the pharmaceutical field. Further, in order to keep the length and size of these reference books within the reasonable limit, some of the information regarding less frequently used drugs/ old monographs or substances which are not currently in practice is omitted in the new/revised editions of the book updated from time to time.

Classification

These standard text/drug-compendia can be classified into *Official compendia and Non-official compendia*

A. *Official Compendia*

Official compendia are the compilations of drugs and other related substances which are recognized as legal standards of purity, quality and strength by a government agency of respective countries of their origin. For example- British Pharmacopoeia (BP), British Pharmaceutical Codex (BPC), Indian Pharmacopoeia (IP), United States Pharmacopoeia (USP), National Formulary (NF), The State Pharmacopoeia of USSR and Pharmacopoeias of other countries

B. *Non-Official Compendia*

The book other than official drug compendia which are used as secondary reference sources for drugs and other related substances are known as non-official drug compendia. *For example*-Merck Index, Extra Pharmacopoeia (Martindale) and United States Dispensatory.

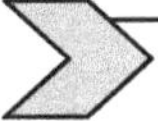 ## Indian Pharmacopoeial Commission (IPC)

IPC (an autonomous institution of the Ministry of health and family welfare, Government of India) was formed according to the Indian Drugs and Cosmetics Act of 1940 and established under the executive orders of the Government of India in 1956, primarily works in close coordination with all the stakeholders (including pharmaceutical industry, drug control laboratories, research and teaching institutions) of Indian Pharmacopoeia (IP) for the development of monographs.

IPC is mandated to set standards of drugs alongwith the updation of such standards of drugs commonly required for treatment of diseases prevailing in this country on regular basis.

IPC publishes official documents for improving quality of medicines by way of adding new and updating existing monographs (encompasses information related to chemical structures of drugs and their properties such as molecular weight, physical description, solubility, identification tests, standards, assay method, storage etc.) It further promotes rational use of generic medicines by publishing National Formulary of India (NFI). IP prescribes standards for identity, purity and strength of drugs essentially required from health care perspective of human beings and animals. IPC also provides IP Reference Substances (IPRS) which act as a finger print for identification of an article under test and its purity as prescribed in IP.

Recently, in 1st of July, 2022, IPC released the 9th edition of 'IP-2022' comprising 3152 monographs. A total of 92 new monographs for drugs have been added to IP 2022 edition. Monographs of *lorcaserin hydrochloride tablets and locraserin hydrochloride hemihydrate* have been omitted form the current IP edition vide IPC's Notice dated March 10, 2021. Further a general chapter on assay of Human Anti-D Immunoglobulin Methods B and C has also been omitted from IP 2022.

Objectives

✓ To develop comprehensive monographs for drugs to be included in the Indian Pharmacopoeia (IP), comprising of active pharmaceutical ingredients, pharmaceutical aids and dosage forms as well as medical devices and to keep them updated by revision on a regular basis.

✓ To develop monographs for herbal drugs, both raw drugs and extracts/formulations there from.

✓ To accord priority to monographs of drugs included in the National Essential Medicines List and their dosage forms.

✓ To take note of the different levels of sophistication in analytical testing/ instrumentation available while framing the monographs.

✓ To accelerate the process of preparation, certification and distribution of IP Reference Substances, including the related substances, impurities and degradation products.

✓ To collaborate with pharmacopoeias like the Ph Eur, BP, USP, JP, ChP and International Pharmacopoeia with a view to harmonizing with global standards.

✓ To review existing monographs periodically with a view to deleting obsolete ones and amending those requiring upgrading /revision.

✓ To organize educational programs and research activities for spreading and establishing awareness on the need and scope of quality standards for drugs and related articles /materials.

✓ To publish the NFI for updating medical practitioners and other healthcare professionals.

✓ To act as a National Coordination Centre for Pharma-covigilance Programme of India.

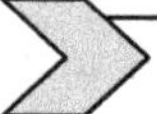 ## The Indian Pharmacopoeia

Some of the earliest reference to the development of pharmacopoeia in India dates back to 1563 and the credit goes to *Garcia da Orta* a Portugese physician-cum-teacher. The first raw form of IP was conceived in 1837 which got actual shape in the form of Bengal Pharmacopoeia and Conspectus of Drugs in 1841.

In 1946, Indian Pharmacopoeial list containing drugs both included (i.e. crude drugs, chemicals and their preparations) and not included (i.e. drugs of plant origin, drugs of animal origin, biological products, insecticides, colouring agents, synthetics, miscellaneous and drugs for veterinary use) in the British Pharmacopoeia along with standards to protect their usefulness, tests for identity and purity was released by Department of Health, Govt. of India under the chairmanship of Col. Sir R.N. Chopra along with other nine members. This Indian Pharmacopoeial list published in 1946 actually laid the foundation of official document in the form of first edition of Indian Pharmacopoeia published in 1955. Further, its draft preparation was initiated in 1944 with directions to Drugs Technical Advisory Board by the Government of India.

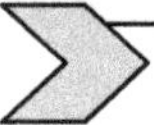

Historical Timeline of IP

Published/ Released by	Time Line	Publication Events
IP Commiteee *(Under the chairmanship of Dr. B.N. Ghosh)*	1946	Release of *Indian Pharmacopoeial List* by GoI
	1948	The GoI constituted a permanent Indian Pharmacopoeia Committee (IPC). and tasked to formulate IP and to keep it up-to-date
	1955	The **1****stedition ofIP**
	1960	Supplement of IP 1955 *(Note-The revision of IP as well as compilation of its new edition was taken up simultaneously by the committee. However, after the death of Dr. B.N..Ghosh in 1958, Dr. B. Mukherjee, the Director of CDRI was appointed as the chairman of IPC.)*
	1966	The **2ndedition of IP**
	1975	Supplement of IP 1966 *(Note- In 1978, The IPC was reconstituted by the GoI, MHFW, under the chairmanship of Dr. Nitya Nand, Director, CDRI, Lucknow)*
	1985	The **3rdedition of IP** in two volumes, Vol.-I & Vol.-II
	1989 &1991	Addendum (I) and (II) to IP 1985 respectively
	1996	The **4thedition of IP**
	2000	Veterinary Supplement
	2000 and 2002	Addendum to IP 1996 respectively
IP Commission	2005	Addendum to IP 1996 respectively
	2007	The **5th edition of IP**
	2008	Addendum to IP
	2010	The **6th edition of IP**
	2012	Addendum to IP
	2014	The **7th edition of IP**
	2015 & 2016	Addendum (I) and (II) to IP 2014 respectively
	2018	The **8th edition of IP with four volumes in DVD as well as hard form**
	2019 & 2021	Addendum (I) and (II) to IP, 2018 respectively
	2022	The **9th edition of IP**

The yearwise addition in the number of new monographs from 1985 to 2022 being depicted in successive IPs indicates the continuous updation in the information related to drugs and medicinal substances.

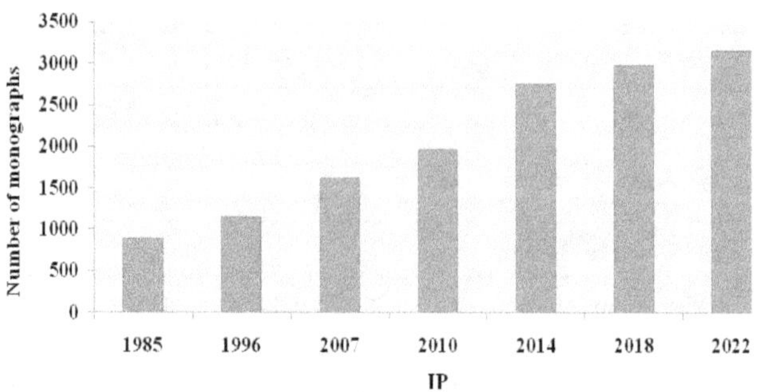

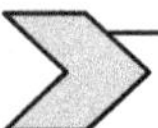 ## Process for IP Monograph Development

People from all segments of pharmaceutical fraternity including public reviews and comments are given special attention while developing the IP standards. The principle of *"openness, justice and fairness"* is kept in mind during compiling and editing the contents of the Indian Pharmacopoeia. Figure below illustrates the methodology adopted for the development of a monograph in I.P.

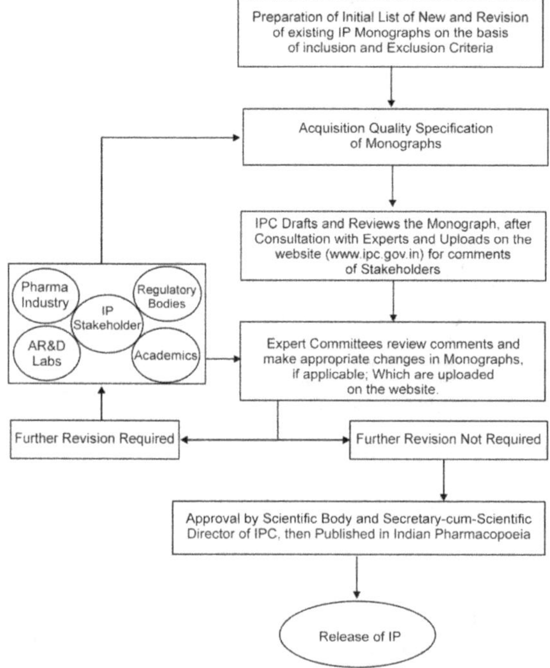

The process of development of a monograph
(Courtesy: https://www.ipc.gov.in)

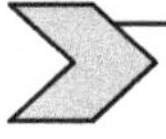 ## Some Other Official Publications Related to Pharmacy Profession in India

National Formulary of India (NFI)

'Formulary' is a manual containing clinically oriented summaries of pharmacological information about selected drugs which serve as a guidance for medical practitioners, medical students, pharmacists in hospitals and different sectors in sales departments. This manual may incorporate administrative and regulatory information pertaining to the prescribing and dispensing of drugs. It also contains information about drug interaction, resistance, cumulative effects, drug dependence, prescription writing etc.

In general, a national formulary focuses on available and cost effective medicines that are relevant to the treatment of diseases, native or endemic to a particular region or a country.

The first NFI was published in 1960 by the Ministry of Health. The second and third formularies were published in 1966 and 1979 respectively. To address the need of publication of an updated version of NFI, Ministry of Health and Family Welfare, Govt. of India vide their Notification No. F.No.X.11035/2/06- DFQC dated 8th May, 2008 assigned this mandatory responsibility to the Indian Pharmacopoeia Commission (IPC), Ghaziabad. Therefore, from 2008 the NFI is published by the Indian Pharmacopoeia Commission on behalf of the Health Ministry. The current edition of NFI-2021 (adopted from the WHO Model Formulary) is presently in use for reference which has been thoroughly updated for its content, especially keeping in view the end user in India and guidance to medical practitioners.

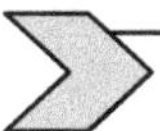 ## Pharmacist's Oath
(Courtesy: Pharmacy Council of India)

I swear by the code of ethics of Pharmacy Council of India, in relation to the community and shall act as an integral part of health care team.

I shall uphold the laws and standards governing my profession.

I shall strive to perfect and enlarge my knowledge to contribute to the advancement of pharmacy and public health.

I shall follow the system which I consider best for Pharmaceutical care and counseling of patients.

I shall endeavor to discover and manufacture drugs of quality to alleviate sufferings of humanity. I shall hold in confidence the knowledge gained about the patients in connection with my professional practice and never divulge unless compelled to do so by the law.

I shall associate with organizations having their objectives for betterment of the profession of Pharmacy and make contribution to carry out the work of those organizations.

While I continue to keep this oath unviolated, may it be granted to me to enjoy life and the practice of pharmacy respected by all, at all times!

Should I trespass and violate this oath, may the reverse be my lot !

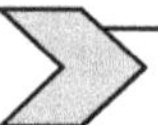

Pharmacist's Code of Ethics
(As adopted by Pharmacy Council of India)

Ethics is defined as 'code of moral principles'. It emphasizes on the determination of right or wrong while doing one's duty. Code of Pharmaceutical Ethics as formulated by Pharmacy Council of India are meant to guide the pharmacist as to how he should conduct himself (or herself), in relation to himself (or herself), his / her patrons (owner of the pharmacy), general public, co-professionals etc. and patients.

Introduction

The profession of pharmacy is noble in its ideals and pious in its character. Apart from being a career for earning livelihood, it has inherent attitude of service and sacrifice in the interests of the suffering humanity. The lofty ideals set up by *Charaka,* the ancient Philosopher, Physician and Pharmacist in his enunciation: *"Even if your own life be in danger you should not betray or neglect the interests of your patients"* should be fondly cherished by all Pharmacists.

A Pharmacist must, above all be a good citizen and must uphold and defend the laws of the state and the Nation.

Government has restricted the practice of Pharmacy to only Professional Pharmacists i.e. Registered Pharmacist under the Pharmacy Act 1948. PCI framed the following ethics for Indian Pharmacists, which may be categorized under the following headings:

✓ Pharmacist in relation to his job.

✓ Pharmacist in relation to his trade.

✓ Pharmacist in relation to medical profession.

✓ Pharmacist in relation to his profession.

Pharmacist in Relation to His Job

A pharmacist should keep the following things in relation to his job.

(i) *Pharmaceutical services*

A Registered pharmacist should provide comprehensive pharmaceutical service (which involves the supply of commonly required medicines without undue delay) and have a willingness to furnish emergency supplies at all times.

(ii) *Conduct of the Pharmacy*

The conditions in a pharmacy should be such as to preclude avoidable risk error of accidental contamination in the preparation, dispensing and supply of medicines. The appearance of the premises should reflect the professional character of the pharmacy. It should be clear to the public that the practice of pharmacy is carried out in the establishment.

(iii) *Handling of Prescription*

When a prescription is presented for dispensing, it should be received by a pharmacist without any discussion or comment over it regarding the merits and demerits of its therapeutic efficiency. In matter of refilling prescriptions, a pharmacist should solely be guided by the instructions of a prescriber and he should advise patients to use medicines or remedies strictly in accordance with the intention of the physician as noted on the prescription.

(iv) *Handling of drugs*

All possible care should be taken to dispense a prescription correctly by weighing and measuring all ingredients in correct proportions by the help of scale and measures. Further, a Pharmacist should always use drugs and medicinal preparations of standard quality available.

(v) *Apprentice Pharmacist*

While in-charge of a dispensary, drug store or hospital pharmacy where apprentice pharmacists are admitted for practical training, a pharmacist should see that the trainees are given full facilities for their work so that on the completion of their training they have acquired sufficient technique and skill to make themselves dependable pharmacists. No certificate or credentials should be granted unless the above criterion is attained and the recipient has proved himself worthy of the same.

Pharmacist in Relation to His Trade

Following are the provisions which pharmacist should keep in mind while dealing with his trade:

(i) *Price structure*

Prices charged from customers should be fair and in keeping with the quality and quantity of commodity supplied and the labor and skill required in making it ready for use, so as to ensure an adequate remuneration to the pharmacist taking into consideration his knowledge, skill, the time consumed and the great responsibility involved, but at the same time without unduly taxing the purchaser.

(ii) *Fair trade practice*

No attempt should be made to capture the business of a contemporary by cut-throat competition, that is, by offering any sort of prizes or gifts or any kind of allurement to patronizes or by knowingly charging lower prices for medical commodities than those charged by a fellow pharmacist if they be reasonable. In case any order or prescription genuinely intended to be served by some dispensary is brought by mistake to another, the latter should refuse to accept it and should direct the customer to the right place. Labels, trademarks and other signs and symbols of contemporaries should not be imitated or copied.

(iii) *Purchase of drugs*

Drugs should always be purchased from genuine and reputable sources and a pharmacist should always be on his guard not to aid or abet, directly or indirectly the manufacture, possession, distribution and sale of spurious or sub-standard drugs.

(iv) *Advertising and Displays*

No display material either on the premises, in the press or elsewhere should be used by a pharmacist in connection with the sale to the public of medicines or medical appliances which is undignified in style.

Pharmacist in Relation to Medical Profession

Following are the code of ethics of a pharmacist in relation to medical profession:

(i) *Limitation of professional activity*

The professional activity of the medical practitioner as well as the pharmacists should be confined to their own field only. Medical practitioners should not possess drugs stores and pharmacists should not diagnose diseases and prescribe remedies. A pharmacist may, however, can deliver first aid to the victim in case of accident or emergency.

(ii) *Cladenstine arrangement*

A pharmacist should not enter into a secret arrangement or contract with a physician by offering him any commission or any advantages.

(iii) *Liasion with public.*

A pharmacist should always maintain proper link between physicians and people. He should advise the physicians on pharmaceutical matters and should educate the people regarding health and hygiene. The pharmacist should be keeping himself / herself up-to-date with pharmaceutical knowledge from various journals or publications. Any information acquired by a pharmacist during his professional activities should not be disclosed to any third party until and unless required to do so by law.

Pharmacist in Relation to His Profession

Regarding to the profession the following code of ethics should be fulfilled.

(i)   *Professional vigilance*

A pharmacist must abide by the pharmaceutical laws and he/she should see that other pharmacists are abiding it.

(ii) *Law-abiding citizens*

The pharmacists should have a fair knowledge of the laws of the country pertaining to food, drug, pharmacy, health, sanitation etc.

(iii) *Relationship with Professional Organizations*

A pharmacist should be actively involved in professional organization, should advance the cause of such organizations.

(iv) *Decorum and Propriety*

A pharmacist should not indulge in doing anything that goes against the decorum and propriety of Pharmacy Profession.

Regulatory Authorities of Different Regions/Countries

1.   **INDIA** – CDSCO (Central drugs standard control organization)
2.   **USA** - FDA (Food & Drug Administration)
3.   **CANADA** – HPFB (Health products & food branch)
4.   **Australia** – TGA (Therapeutic goods administration)
5.   **JAPAN** – PFSB (Pharmaceutical & food safety bureau), PMDA (Pharmaceutical & medical devices agency)
6.   **CHINA** – NMPA (National medical products administration)
7.   **EUROPE** – EMA (European medicines agency)
8.   **RUSSIA** – Ministry of health of the Russian federation

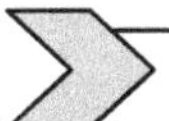

Good Dispensing Practice (GDP) Guidelines
(As recommended by World Health Organization)

Good Dispensing Practice (GDP) warrants that the right medicines of desired quality are delivered fittingly to the right patient with the right dose, strength, frequency, dosage form and quantity, together with clear instructions, both written and verbal and with appropriate packaging suitable for maintaining the quality and efficacy of the medicine. A safe, clean and organized working environment provides the basis for GDP.

The dispensing environment includes:
➢ Qualified / trained staff Appropriate physical surroundings
➢ Adequate shelving and storage areas
➢ Proper work surfaces

➢ Suitable equipment

➢ Necessary packaging materials

Scope: The scope and application of GDP guidelines is pertinent to only:

- Poisons list of substances (as per WHO)
- Medicines for human use
- Public healthcare facilities
- Licensed private healthcare facilities (clinics, hospitals, community pharmacies, dental clinics)

Dispensing Process

Adherence to good dispensing procedures is vital in ensuring that medicines are dispensed correctly and any potential/ real errors which may occur during the dispensing process are detected and rectified before medicines reach the patient.

Who should be involved in the process of dispensing?

(a) Screening of Prescription: Healthcare professional (Registered medical practitioner/ registered dentist/ pharmacist)

(b) Preparation of Medicines: Pharmacist, registered medical practitioner or a person under immediate supervision of a pharmacist/ medical practitioner

(c) Supplying the Medicines: Registered medical practitioner, registered dentist or pharmacist

(d) Counseling: By healthcare professional

General instructions for Students in a Practical Dispensing Lab

✓ Each student is expected to work on his/her own. If advice is needed, it should be obtained only from the class teacher conducting practical lab or a lab technician.

✓ Each student should have a duster cloth or small hand towel, a pair of scissors, a pair of forceps, a pair of scapula, a set of pencil colours, a black/blue pen and red pen (fine point), a ruler and a calculator.

✓ Each student should possess a dispensable paper towels at the end of each bench/slab for mopping up wet spillage if occurs. All work for dispensing the dosage form should be conducted in a clean and tidy manner.

✓ Read the prescription/composition/formula for the dosage form or pill carefully, if necessary verify the composition from most recent editions of I.P. or B.P. or U.S.P. or Martindale.

✓ The student should work out the amount to be used from the formula and write them in ink after checking the calculations in two ways if possible.

- ✓ In pharmaceutical calculations, the student should always have the habit of protecting the decimal point with a '0' i.e. 0.1 not .1; since if the decimal point is not written distinctly, there is a risk of administrating/prescribing a ten times (×10) overdose.

- ✓ The student must always write down the details of every weighing and measurement.

- ✓ Every student should possess pre-calibrated weights before any manual weighing procedure with precision and accuracy and cross contamination of products or excipients should be avoided at any cost.

- ✓ The student should exercise care while considering approximations. In general, it should not be made when the amount is being weighed or measured with the weights. Unless it is unavoidable, try to add minimal approximations (or NMT 5%). Further, the student must write the correct amount first and show the approximation in brackets at the side – e.g. 12.678g (12.68g).

- ✓ The student must use a spatula for weighing solids. This avoids fouling the neck of the bottle. In order to keep out the dust, the student should hold the bottle as near to horizontal as possible with one hand and remove the stopper with the little finger and palm of the other. Unless the stopper is too large, keep it in the hand; the student will find that he/she can easily use the spatula with the same hand. If it is essential to put the stopper down, place it the right way up on a clean sheet of white paper.

- ✓ The student must look up for the storage requirements of the preparation or the medicaments if the preparation is a special formulation not prescribed in one of these standard books (i.e. I.P./U.S.P./B.P.). Choose the correct container for storage, protection from light, storage in a cool place, etc. may also be necessary.

- ✓ After finalizing the preparation, store the product into the container and the preparation must be protected from accidental contamination.

- ✓ For liquids to be transferred, the student should hold the bottle in such a way that the label is on the opposite side. This will prevent the label from getting spoilt while transferring the liquid.

- ✓ No ingredient should be transferred and kept on paper to ensure its identity till the end.

- ✓ *Labelling:* The student should cut the label to fit the container but do not trim off the name of the preparation or the supplier (the manufacturing group). Use the largest possible label on the dosage form.

- ✓ During the labelling procedure, if a wrong figure or unit is written, cross it out and write the correct one above of at the side. But don't overwrite it or alter the wrong one.

✓ The student must carefully observe the labels of the stock bottles while using and watch particularly for words such as Compound (e.g. Compound tragacanth powder is different from tragacanth powder); concentration (e.g. Concentrated compound infusion of Gentianis different from Compound Infusion of Gentian); Strong (Fort)(e.g. Strong Coal Tar Solution is different from Coal tar solution). Moreover, the student must be vigilant for medicaments that have similar names (e.g. Eucalyptol and Eucalyptus oil) or e.g. Terebone and Turpentine Oil (Oil Terebinth).

✓ The student should check the label of the stock bottle against the composition formula before and after using the prescription.

✓ The student should hold the bottle with the label uppermost so that it can be seen during use. As a result, an error may be detected. Also, liquid from the rim will not run down the label.

✓ ***Presentation of the Label after dosage form design:*** The student should receive or get issued the clean and polished glass or plastic containers from the store keeper. Polishing should be done after, as well as before labelling, to remove gum and finger- marks.

✓ Acacia-gum labels will not adhere to plastics or metal containers; self-adhesive labels must be used.

How to Write a Dosage Form Design Experiment in a Note Book
(Left Side Page of the Notebook)

Step 1: Write 'AIM OF THE EXPERIMENT' on the left side page of the practical note book and record the date on the right side of the note book

Step 2: Write the material/chemical and equipment requirements as per the requirement of the experiment.

Step 3: Write the exact 'CHEMICAL FORMULA' of the dosage form or prescription as written depicting all the names and record the quantity of each ingredient/substance in a tabular form opposite the name of the drug to which it refers.

Step 3: Check for the prescription/dosage form refers to I.P., NFI., U.S.P., B.P., B.P.C., or B.N.F. preparation, and record the official formula together with the official quantities, and record as in the quantities used.

Step 4: *Calculation of doses:* Calculate and Convert the prescription composition or chemical formula of the dosage form indicating all the ingredients as per the dispensing amount of the experiment and record the details of all calculations of doses and quantities for dilutions and trituration for each active ingredient.

Step 5: Design a 'SPECIMEN LABEL' using example as shown below on the left side page of your note book

<table>
<tr><td colspan="3" align="center">SIMPLE SYRUP (I.P.) 30 g</td></tr>
<tr>
<td>Composition:
Each 30 g contains:

Oil of peppermint- 0.1 ml
Distilled water q.s.- 50 ml

Dose: 10 to 40 ml

Storage: Store in well-closed,
light-resistant container cool
place to volatilization of oil</td>
<td>SHERRICOF®
(Simple Syrup)

(Used as an antispasmodic
and carminative in flatulence
of the gastrointestinal tract,
cramping and bloating,
flatulent colic to relieve
nausea and vomiting, and as a
gentle aromatic stimulant)

PROTECT FROM SUN
LIGHT
NOT FOR INJECTION</td>
<td>Mfg. Lic. No.- HAT/2018
Batch No.- AKH 4311
Mfg. Date- Jan. 2018
Exp. Date- Dec. 2019
M.R.P.- Rs. 49.00
(Inclusive of all taxes)

Mfd. By: AKT
PHARMA
SADIQ ROAD,
PATIALA
PB-147002</td>
</tr>
</table>

Step 6: Affix a duplicate of the label applied to the product and include also any auxiliary labels used; e.g. shake the bottle well before use (if required).

Step 7: *Container:* Record details of the size and type of container used together with any special container specification for the product. E.g. test for the limit of alkalinity of glass (L.A.G.).

Step 8: *Storage Requirements:* Record the shelf life of the product and details of any special requirements for storage, e.g. Protect from light.

(Right Side Page of the Notebook)

Step 1: Write 'AIM OF THE EXPERIMENT' at the top as heading on the right side page of the practical note book and record the date on the right side of the note book.

Step 2: Write the 'REFERNCE' from a standard compendia or text book source or practical manual from where the composition or formula of the prescription/ dosage form was taken in a following manner:

(Full surname with first name in abbreviated form, title of the chapter, In: (title of the book/journal), Editors name, Publishers name, Chapter number, issue and volume of the book, year of 0publication)

Step 3: THEORY: *Main pharmaceutical actions of the active drug/ excipients:* Write a brief account on the main pharmaceutical actions of the active ingredients in the preparation, in the context of the dosage form supplied.

Clinical Conditions and Dose Regimen of Product: It has to be noted that this action refers to the final dispensed product only, and not to other dosage forms of the same drugs.

Step 4:   METHODS OF PREPARATION: A detailed description of the step wise procedure or in a note form with every possible details used in the methods. (Note-*Clarification: Wherever applicable, specify the medium used; Sterlization: Wherever applicable, specify the record methods, time and temperature). Formulation notes-* Record the details of additives, excipients, colouring agents and aids used in the dosage form design. Mention also any incompatibilities encountered. If you have formulated the product, give the reasons for your choice of formulation.

Step 5:   GENERAL PRECAUTIONS:

- Verify the doses of internal preparations (including suppositories and enemas) and take into account the directions for use.

- In case of any over dosage, report to the lab technician or class incharge.

- If any ingredient used in the chemical formula belongs to the category of a poison (or mentioned in the Poisons and T.S.A. Guide or mentioned on the label of the stock bottle/container) the weight or volume must be dispensed by the lab technician or Class incharge only.

- In order to confirm if there is no pharmaceutical or pharmacological incompatibility, use I.P., B.P., U.S.P or Extra Pharmacopoeia. In case of any doubt about the method of preparation, refer to previous dispensing schedules.

- Step 6: RESULTS: Report the inference or conclusion of the experiment in a one line only.(*Note: The experiment should be reported on the index page of the note book and get it signed from the class incharge after the viva-voce of the experiment)*

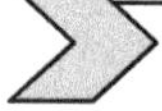

General Packaging Instructions for Dispensing

Packaging Instructions:

The choice of container used for dispensing medicines for the packaging of individual preparations is made solely on technical grounds. Official recommendations on colours and changes of container for each type of medication should be adhered, so as to reduce the accidental misuse of medicines. The following points are to be noted in the packaging of dispensed products.

- All mixtures intended for oral use must be packed in plain bottles and covered with plastic screw-caps.
- All preparations intended for external use only (e.g. Gargles, lotions, etc.) must be packed in fluted or ribbed glass bottles.
- All preparations containing photo-labile (i.e. light-sensitive) ingredients are packed in amber coloured bottles.
- Any thick liquid preparations such as emulsion, liniments etc. are packed in wide-mouthed bottles to allow for easy pouring out of contents from the bottle.

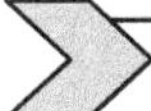 ## Labeling Directions for Various Types of Preparations

Aim of the Labeling:

The primary aim of any label is to accurately direct the patient as to how and when the medicine should be taken or used. Therefore, a label is an important factor in the appearance of the final medicine and a high standard in label presentation that will do much to maintain confidence of the patient. Hence, every effort should be made to be competent on this point.

In nutshell, the mantra for an ideal label should be

'LEGIBLE, NEAT AND WELL-BALANCED'

General Instructions:

Choose the correct size of container for the product and match the label size to the container.

✓ Polish the bottles or containers before labeling.

✓ Affix labels symmetrically on the container.

✓ Never have more than one unlabelled product on the bench at the same time.

✓ Never place a fresh label over an old label which may pose dangerous hazards.

✓ Generally, labels for 'Internal Medicines' adopt black prints and those for 'External Medicines' adopt red prints.

✓ The main label should clearly state the quantity of the product, the type of preparation e.g. 'The Mixture' 'The Tablets', etc. or where so directed the actual name of the preparation.

✓ In a case if any official (I.P., N.F.I., U.S.P., B.P., or Extra Pharmacopoeia) dosage form is being dispensed, it is not necessary to declare on the label, the concentration of the active ingredients. It is for instance sufficient to label the product as, 'AMMONIUM CHLORIDE AND MORPHINE MIXTURE BP 188. Vol.I.'

✓ Write precise instructions for use in minimum words. Add the date of dispensing and a reference number (if it is a private prescription),the name of the patient, the name and address of the pharmacy. (*Note- The word 'POISON' should not appear on the label of a dispensed medicine unless specifically requested*)

For some preparations, instructions which are specifically detailed on the prescription must be given on the container. Such instructions serve to amplify how the medicine is to be used or to guide the patient regarding the best storage conditions. Auxiliary labels should be sensibly positioned relative to the main label and should not be fixed on the main label.

Auxiliary label	Circumstances in which label is used	Examples of preparations for which the label is appropriate
SHAKE THE BOTTLE	Liquid preparations which are disperse systems	Emulsions and Suspensions
	Liquid preparations where precipitations or separation is considered possible	
FOR EXTERNAL USE ONLY	Liquid preparations for external application Solid and semi-solid preparations for external application	Lotions, liniments, skin paints Creams, dusting powders and ointments
NOT TO BE TAKEN ORALLY (A possible alternative label for these products)	Liquid preparation which are not administered orally and which are not applied to a skin surface	Ear Drops, eye Lotions, eye Drops, Inhalations, nasal drops, enemas
NOT TO BE TAKEN BY MOUTH	Solid dosage forms which might inadvertently be administered by oral route	Inhalation, pessaries, some solutions, tablets for external use, and suppositories

Some Important Pharmacopoeial Definitions

Temperature

STORAGE CONDITION (I.P)	TEMPERATURE (ºC)
Cold	2-8
Cool	8-25
Warm	30-40
Excess heat	> 40

Volume Measure

MEASURE OF LIQUID TRANSFERRED (U.S.P)	VOLUME IN METRIC SYSTEM (ml)	VOLUME IN IMPERIAL SYSTEM
One drop	0.06	1 minim
One teaspoonful	5.0	1 fluid drachm
One dessertspoonful	8.0	2 fluid drachm
One tablespoonful	15.0	0.5 fluid ounce
One wineglassful	60.0	2 fluid ounce
One teacupful	120.0	4 fluid ounce
One tumblerful	240.0	8 fluid ounce

Powders (I.P.)

CLASSIFICATION	DESIGNATION	DEFINITION
Coarse powder	10/44	A powder of which all particles pass through a sieve no. 10 and not more than 40% by weight pass through sieve no. 44
Moderately coarse powder	22/60	A powder of which all particles pass through a sieve no. 22 and not more than 40% by weight pass through sieve no. 60
Moderately fine powder	44/85	A powder of which all particles pass through a sieve no. 44 and not more than 40% by weight pass through sieve no. 85
Fine powder	85/120	A powder of which all particles pass through a sieve no. 85 and not more than 40% by weight pass through sieve no. 120
Very fine powder	120/350	A powder of which all particles pass through a sieve no. 120 and not more than 40% by weight pass through sieve no. 350
Micro fine powder	350	A powder of which not less than 90% by weight of the particles pass through a sieve no. 350
Superfine powder	--	A powder of which not less than 90% by number of the particles are less than 10 micron in size

CLASSIFICATION OF DOSAGE FORMS

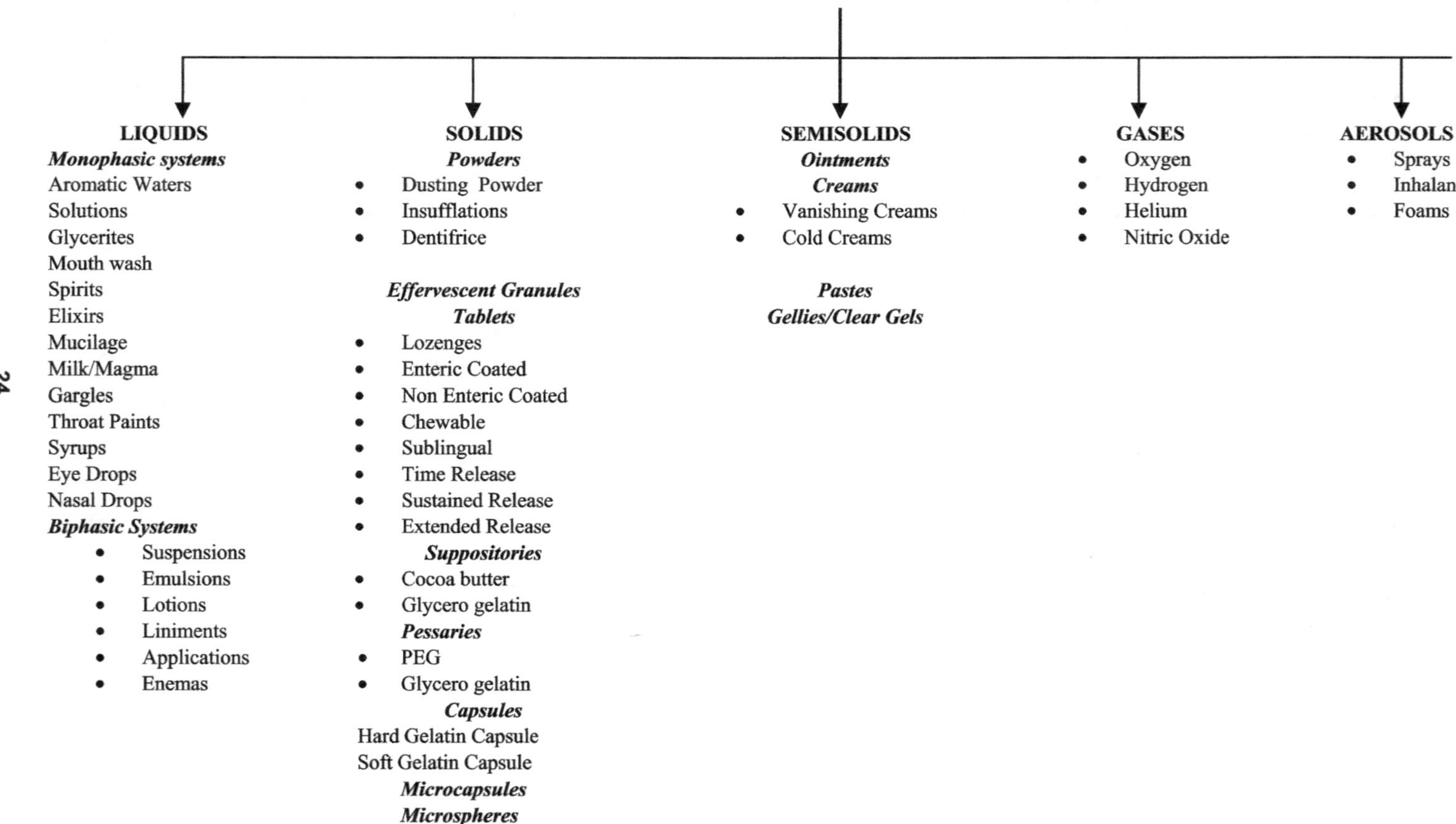

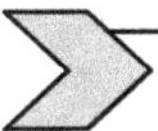

Routes of Drug Administration

A drug will produce its action only when it enters the body, tissue or cells (i.e. site of action). So the entrance through which a drug is delivered is called the route of drug administration.

Classification

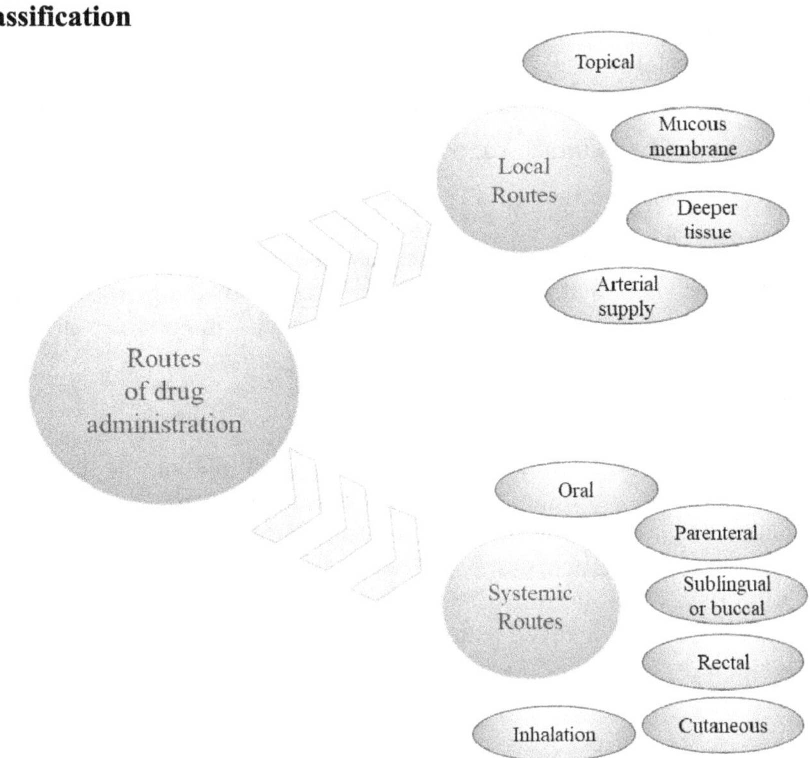

Local Routes

These routes can only be used for localized lesions at accessible sites. Systemic absorption of the drug from these routes is minimal or absent. Thus, high concentrations are attained at the desired site without exposing the rest of the body.

Topical

This refers to external application of the drug to the surface for localized action.

(a) **Skin:** Drug is applied as ointment, cream, lotion, paste, powder, dressing etc.

(b) **Mucous membrane:** The dosage form depends on the site:

    ✓ *Mouth and pharynx:* Paints, lozenges, mouth washes, gargles.

✓ *Eyes, ears and nose:* Drops, ointments, irrigation, nasal spray.

✓ *Gastrointestinal tract:* Non-absorbable drugs given orally e.g. aluminum hydroxide, magnesium hydroxide, methyl polysiloxane etc.

✓ *Bronchi and lungs*: As inhalations, aerosols (nebulized solution or fine powder)- e.g. salbutamol, cromolyn sodium.

✓ *Urethra:* Jellies e.g. lidocaine, irrigating solutions.

✓ *Vagina:* Pessaries, vaginal tablets, inserts, cream, powders, douches.

✓ *Anal canal:* Ointment, suppositories.

Deeper Tissues

Certain deep areas can be approached by using a syringe and needle, but the drug should be such that systemic absorption is slow. e.g. intra-articular injection (hydrocortisone acetate), intra-thecal injection (lidocaine, amphotericin B) and retrobulbar injection (xylocaine).

Arterial Supply

Close intra-arterial injection is used for contrast media in femoral or bronchial artery for limb malignancies. In these cases, the drug is injected into the artery that is supplying the blood to the desired site (i.e., site for diagnosis or the cancerous tissues). The drug travels with the blood flow towards the tissue it is perfusing and not towards the heart. Thus, systemic action is avoided and localized action is achieved. (*Note - In case of vein the drug will be carried to the heart and from there to the system i.e. to the whole body*).

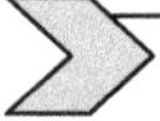 **Systemic Routes**

Parenteral

(*Par-* beyond, *enteral-* intestinal). Routes of drug administration other than oral route are known as parenteral route. This refers to administration by injection which takes the drug directly into the tissue fluid or blood without having to cross the intestinal mucosa and subsequently liver.

Advantages: Absorption is faster, hence drug can be administered rapidly and in accurate dose in time of emergencies.

✓ Gastric irritation and vomiting are avoided.

✓ It can be employed in unconscious, uncooperative or vomiting patients.

✓ There are no chances of interference by food or digestive juices.

✓ Liver is bypassed.

Diverse systemic routes which are intended for the administration of drug to be absorbed into blood and distributed all over, including the site of action, through circulation.

Systemic Routes	Enteral								Parenteral			
	Oral	Sublingual /buccal	Rectal	Cutaneous	Inhala Tional	Intra-peritoneal	Intra—arterial	Nasal	IV	IM	SC	ID
Mode	Dosage form is taken through the mouth and it is absorbed from the GIT	Dosage form is placed under the tongue (sublingual) or crushed in the mouth and spread over the buccal mucosa. The drug is absorbed through the buccal mucosa	Drug containing dosage form is either inserted or put into the rectum as suppositories or retention enema. One part of the absorbed drug passes to the liver, another part to the systemic circulation	Dosage form is applied or placed on the skin and the drug penetrates the skin to reach the blood i.e. cutaneous route is meant for systemic absorption.	The drug is administered through nose or mouth, carried by the air to reach the lung. The alveoli are rich with capillary vessels. The drug is diffused into the blood stream. Thus systemic action is obtained	Drug is injected into the peritoneal cavity.	Drug is injected into an artery. The effect of a drug can be localized in a particular organ or tissue by choosing the appropriate artery	Drug is administered as snuff or spray or nebulized solution in the nose; where the drug penetrates the nasal mucous membrane to reach the blood	Drug is injected as a bolus or infused slowly over hours in one of the superficial veins (generally brachial vein).	Drug is injected in one of the large skeletal muscles such as deltoid, triceps, gluteus maximus, rectus femoris	Drug is injected under the skin. The drug is deposited in the loose SC tissue which is richly supplied by nerves (irritant drugs cannot be injected but is less vascular (absorption is slower)	Drug is injected into the dermis of skin raising a bleb (e.g. BCG vaccine, sensitivity testing of drugs) or scarring / multiple puncture of the epidermis through a drop of the drug (small pox vaccine) is done. This route is employed for specific purpose only
Dosage forms	e.g. Solid dosage forms (e.g. tablets, capsules, powders) and liquid dosage forms (e.g elixirs, syrups, emulsions, mixtures)	e.g. Tablets or pellets of Nitroglycerine, isoprenaline, clonidine, nifedipine.	e.g. Aminophylline, indomethacin, paraldehyde, diazepam, ergotamine	e.g. Transdermal patches of nitroglycerin, hyoscine, clonidine and estradiol.E.g. Transdermal drug delivery systems of timolol, testosterone, nicotine and isosorbide dinitrite	e.g. Volatile liquids and gases are given by inhalation- such as general anaesthetics, amylnitrite	e.g. Fluids like glucose and saline can be given to children.	e.g. anti cancer drugs	e.g. Posterior pituitary powder and desmop-ressin powder		e.g. Low volume injections - Vitamin A, hydrocortisone acetate, tetanus toxoid, antibiotic etc.		

Contd....

	Enteral							Parenteral				
Systemic Routes	Oral	Sublingual /buccal	Rectal	Cutaneous	Inhala Tional	Intra-peritoneal	Intra-arterial	Nasal	IV	IM	SC	ID
Pros	More safer, and convenient. No assistance is required for administration. It is painless. The medicament need not be sterile and so is cheaper.	Absorption is relatively rapid - action can be produced in a minute. One can spit the drug after the desired effect has been obtained. The liver is bypassed and drugs with high first-pass metabolism can be absorbed directly into the systemic circulation	Drugs having bad taste or odour can be given through this route. Drug that degrades in acidic pH of the gastric juice can be given through this route. This route can also be used when the patient is having recurrent vomiting.	Highly lipid soluble drugs can be applied over the skin for slow and prolonged absorption. The liver is bypassed through this route. The drug can be incorporated in an ointment and applied over specified area of skin. Transdermal drug delivery systems deliver the drug in a controlled manner and for a prolonged period. They provide smooth plasma concentration of drug.	Absorption takes place from the vast surface of alveoli - hence action is very rapid. When administration is discontinued the drug diffuses back and is rapidly eliminated in expired air. Thus controlled administration is possible with time to time adjustment. Bypasses the liver			The drug can avoid digestive juices and liver. Drugs are readily absorbed from this route.	The drug directly reaches the blood stream and effect is produced immediately, hence, this route can be used in emergencies. The inside of the veins is insensitive and drug gets diluted with blood quickly, therefore, even highly irritant drugs can be given by i.v route. Large volumes can be infused (e.g. normal saline). It is useful in unconscious patients.	Muscle is less richly supplied with sensory nerves, hence mild irritants can be injected. Muscle is more vascular hence absorption is faster than subcutaneous route. It is less painful. Depot preparations can be injected by this route and the action of the drug may be prolonged.	Self injection is possible because deep penetration is not required. Oily solutions or aqueous suspensions can form a depot which will release drug slowly for a prolonged period.	

Contd.....

Systemic Routes	Enteral								Parenteral			
	Oral	*Sublingual /buccal*	*Rectal*	*Cutaneous*	*Inhala Tional*	*Intra– peritoneal*	*Intra– arterial*	*Nasal*	*IV*	*IM*	*SC*	*ID*
Cons	Action is slower and not suitable for emergencies. Unpalatable drugs are difficult to administer. May cause nausea and vomiting (e.g. emetine). Certain drugs are not absorbed (e.g. streptomycin). Some drugs are destroyed by digestive juices (e.g. penicillin G, insulin) or in liver (e.g., nitroglycerin, testosterone, lidocaine)	Only lipid soluble and non-irritating drugs can be administered in this way; Drugs with bad taste or objectionable odour are not possible to administer on the tongue.	Administration of drug through this route is rather inconvenient and embarrassing. Absorption is slower, irregular and often unpredictable. Drug absorbed into external haemorrhoidal veins (about 50%) bypasses liver, but not that absorbed into internal haemorrhoidal veins. Rectal inflammation ca results from highly irritant drugs.	Absorption is very slow. So it cannot be used in emergency situation. Water soluble drugs are minimally absorbed through the skin.	Irritant vapors (ether) cause inflammation of respiratory tract and increase secretion.			Not suitable for irritant drugs	Drugs that precipitate in the blood cannot be administered. Only aqueous solution can be administered. If the needle puncture the vessel (i.e. extra vasation) then thrombo-phlebitis of the injected vein and necrosis of the adjoining tissues may occur. No drug can be given in depot form - so the action is not prolonged compared to other parenteral administrations. Untoward reactions if occur are immediate. Once administered, withdrawal of the drug is not possible.	Since deep penetration is needed hence self-medication is not possible. Large volume cannot be given.	Since skin is richly supplied by nerve-endings hence irritant drugs cannot be injected. This route should be avoided in shock patients.e.g. Insulin injection.	

Disadvantages:

✓ The preparation has to be sterilized and is costlier.

✓ Injection are painful.

✓ Self medication is difficult - another trained person is required to give the injection.

✓ Abscess and inflammation at the site of injection may take place.

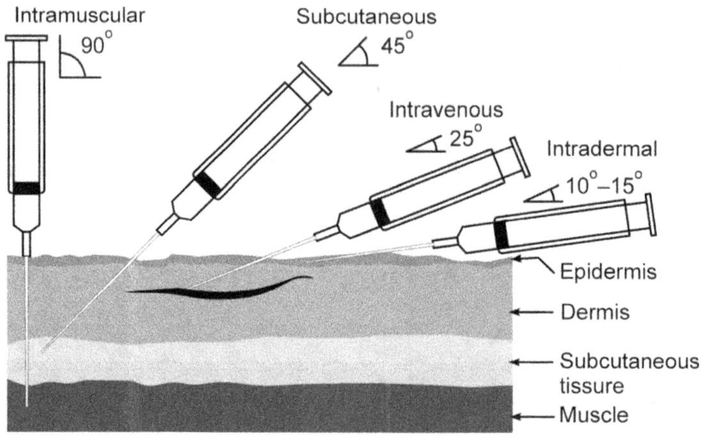

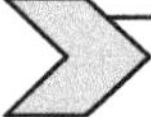 **Pharmaceutical Terms**

Pharmacokinetics is the subject that deals with 'what body does to the drug'.

This subject includes absorption, distribution, metabolism and excretion of the drugs. It determines the routes of administration, dose, onset of action, time of peak action, duration of action and frequency of administration.

Pharamcodynamics is the subject that deals with 'what drug does to the body'.

It is the study of the effect of drug on the body, its mechanism of action, dose-effect relationship, drug-drug interaction, and factors modifying drug action

Dose is the quantity of a drug to be administered at one time to achieve a therapeutic response.

e.g. Oral adult dose of paracetamol is 325 mg.

Dosage is the determination and regulation of the size (dose), frequency, and number of doses.

e.g. Oral adult dosage of paracetamol is 325 mg thrice a day (t.i.d).

Therapeutic index (or Therapeutic ratio)

By this term the therapeutic effect and untoward effect of a drug is compared. The untoward effect is expressed by TD_{50} i.e toxic dose for 50% animals and the therapeutic effect by ED_{50} i.e. effective dose for 50% of animals.

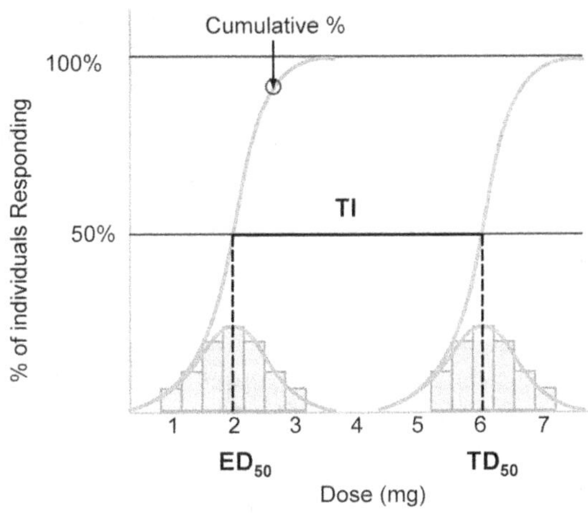

The *therapeutic index* (T.I.) expressed as the ratio of TD_{50} / ED_{50} in humans.

(*Note- Therapeutic index (T.I.) is also expressed as the ratio of LD_{50} / ED_{50} in animals*).

When the therapeutic index is small the drug should be administered under careful observation because the probability of occurance of toxic effect is higher. When the therapeutic effect is large it is safer to administer the drug than with smaller therapeutic index.

The therapeutic index varies widely among substances, even within a related group. For instance, the opioid pain killer remifentanil is very forgiving, offering a therapeutic index of 33,000:1, while Diazepam, a benzodiazepine sedative-hypnotic and skeletal muscle relaxant, has a less forgiving therapeutic index of 100:1. Morphine is even less so with a therapeutic index of 70.

Less safe are cocaine (a stimulant and local anaesthetic) and ethanol (colloquially, the "alcohol" in alcoholic beverages, a widely available sedative consumed worldwide): the therapeutic indices for these substances are 15:1 and 10:1, respectively.

Even less safer drugs such as digoxin, a cardiac glycoside; its therapeutic index is approximately 2:1.

Other examples of drugs with a narrow therapeutic range, which may require drug monitoring both to achieve therapeutic levels and to minimise toxicity, include: paracetamol (acetaminophen), dimercaprol, theophylline, warfarin and lithium carbonate.

Some antibiotics and antifungals require monitoring to balance efficacy with minimising adverse effects, including: gentamicin, vancomycin, amphotericin B (nicknamed 'amphoterrible' for this very reason), and polymyxin B

E.g. benzodiazepines have greater therapeutic index than barbiturates, hence, are less likely to be fatal when taken in accidental overdose.

LD_{50}

Before any new drug molecule is approved for testing in man, extensive toxicity testing is done in various animal species. The crudest type of toxicity test is the LD_{50}.

LD_{50} is defined as the lethal dose for 50% of a group of animals. In other words, it is an individual dose required to kill 50% of test population (i.e. rat, fish, mice, cockroach). Therefore, lower is the LD_{50}, more will be the toxicity of drug/test chemical substance. (For example- A test compound with an LD_{50} value of 10 mg/kg is ten times more toxic than a chemical with LD_{50} value of 100 mg/kg).

Application:-It is used as a standard to compare the relative toxicities of the chemicals

Methods of determination

Various doses of drugs are administered to groups of 10 animals. The mortality (death) in each group within a fixed period of time (say 2 days) is determined and used to construct a curve relating fraction mortality to log (dose).

Significance: It is a parameter which defines (though not adequately) the chemical toxicity of a drug molecule.

Relation of Toxicity with LD_{50}

S.No.	Toxicity	LD_{50} (mg/kg/b.wt.)	Lethal dose	Examples
1.	Super	<0.01	Less than 1 drop	Dioxin; botulism; mushrooms
2.	Extreme	<5	Less than 7 drops	Heroin; nicotine
3.	Very	5-50	7 drops to 1 tsp.	Morphine; codeine
4.	Toxic	50-500	1tsp.	DDT, H_2SO_4; Caffeine
5.	Moderate	500-5K	1oz.-1pt.	Aspirin; wood alcohol
6.	Slightly	5K-15K	1pt.	Ethyl alcohol; soaps
7.	Non-toxic	>15K	>1qt.	Water; table sugar

Protective Index (P.I)

It is a similar concept, except that it uses TD_{50} (median toxic dose) in place of LD_{50}. For many substances, toxic effects can occur at levels far below those needed to cause death, and thus the P.I. (if toxicity is properly specified) is often more informative about a substance's relative safety. Nevertheless, the T.I. is still useful as it can be considered an upper bound for the protective index, and the former also has the advantages of objectivity and easier comprehension.

Therapeutic Window

Also known as pharmaceutical window of a drug, it is the range of drug dosages which can treat disease effectively without having toxic effects. Drugs with a small therapeutic window must be administered with care and control, frequently measuring blood concentration of the drug, to avoid harm. Drugs with narrow therapeutic windows include theophylline, digoxin, lithium, and warfarin.*(Note-Students must take care while using the terms therapeutic index and therapeutic window as both these terms are totally different from each other).*

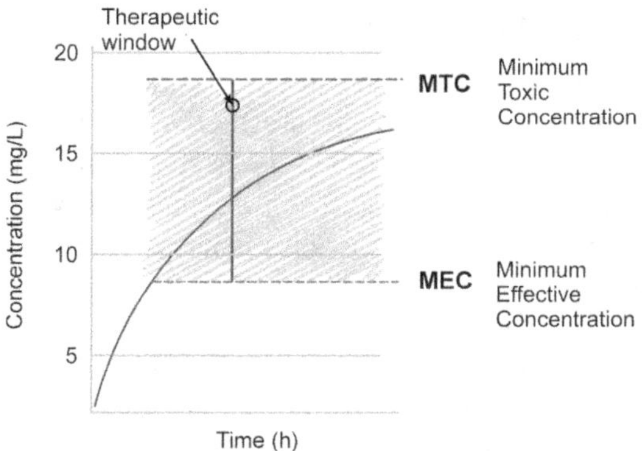

Optimal biological dose (OBD)

The quantity of a drug that will most effectively produce the desired effect while remaining in the range of acceptable toxicity.

Some other terms which are commonly used in relation to expression of doses are:

❖ **Minimum dose**

The lowest dose exerting the desired therapeutic effect in an average patient is said to be a minimum dose. The response of the patient will indicate whether in continuing treatment this dose should be maintained or increased.

❖ **Maximum dose**

The highest dose usually tolerated without undesirable effects in the average patient. This dose is not the greatest amount that can be administered, as in certain specific treatments the official maximum dose may be exceeded.

❖ **Prophylactic dose**

The dose necessary to prevent the onset of a disease

❖ **Therapeutic dose**

The dose necessary to treat an established disease

❖ **Loading dose**

A dose higher than the maintenance, given on the initiation of therapy to give rapid drug plasma levels equivalent to that reached after multiple dosing. This higher dosage is used for a short period of time only; often it only involves a single dose.

❖ **Maintenance dose**

A dose given to maintain the therapeutic level of a drug in the body

❖ **Toxic dose**

The dose capable of producing marked functional derangement in the body.

❖ **Lethal dose**

The smallest dose known to have produced a human death

❖ **Maximum tolerated dose (MTD)**

This refers to the highest dose of a radiological or pharmacological treatment that will produce the desired effect without unacceptable toxicity. The purpose of administering MTD is to determine whether long-term exposure to a chemical might lead to unacceptable adverse health effects in a population, when the level of exposure is not sufficient to cause premature mortality due to short-term toxic effects. The maximum dose is used, rather than a lower dose, to reduce the number of test subjects (and, among other things, the cost of testing), to detect an effect that might occur only rarely. MTD is an essential aspect of a drug's profile and studies are also done in clinical trials. All modern healthcare systems dictate a maximum safe dose for each drug, and generally have numerous safeguards to prevent the prescription and dispensing of quantities exceeding the highest dosage which has been demonstrated to be safe for members of the general patient population.

ED_{50}

There are two type of ED_{50} with which normally the dose effect relationship of a drug is related.

(i)   *50% Effective dose* or *Individual ED_{50}* and;

(ii) *Median effective dose*

(i)   **50% Effective dose (ED_{50})**

In order to have dose-effect relationship the *intensity* of biological effect of a drug is plotted against the *dose* [or log (dose)] of the drug.

Individual ED_{50} is the dose required to elicit 50% of the maximum intensity of the biological effect.

Individual ED_{50} is required to compare the effect between two drugs in an individual.

The *relative potency* of any drug may be obtained by dividing the ED_{50} of the standard, or prototype drug by the drug in question. Since dose-intensity curve varies from individual to individual, hence individual *ED_{50}* is not accurate enough.

(ii) Median effective dose

In this case % of animals showing a desired level of effect is plotted against log (dose) (i.e. *dose-frequency relationship*). The curves generally produced are sigmoidal in nature.

ED_{50} is the dose at which 50% of the animal shows the desired level of effect.

Safety Ratio

Sometimes the term safety ratio is used instead, particularly when referring to psychoactive drugs used for non-therapeutic purposes, e.g. recreational use. In such cases, the effective dose is the amount and frequency that produces the desired effect, which can vary, and can be greater or less than the therapeutically effective dose.

Certain Safety factor (CSF) or Margin of Safety (MOS)

It is the ratio of the lethal dose to 1% of population to the effective dose to 99% of the population (LD_1/ED_{99}). This is a better safety index than the LD_{50} for materials that have both desirable and undesirable effects, because it factors in the ends of the spectrum where doses may be necessary to produce a response in one person but can, at the same dose, be lethal in another.

Special Instructions for Particular Dosage Form

Dosage form	Latin term	Commonly used instructions
Capsules	*Capsula*	*Swallow with a draught of water.*
Creams	*Cremor*	*For external use only.* *Keep in a cool place.*
Dusting powder	*Pulvis*	*For external use only.* *Not to be applied to open wounds or weeping surfaces.*
Ear drops	*Auristillae*	*For external use only.*
Emulsions	*Emulsion*	*Shake the bottle before use.*

Contd...

Dosage form	Latin term	Commonly used instructions
Enemas	*Enema*	*For rectal use only.* *Warm to body temperature before use.*
Eye drops	*Guttae*	*To be used within 30 days after first opening.*
Gargles and mouthwashes	*Gargarisma and Collutrorium*	*Not to be swallowed in large amount.*
Linctuses	*Linctus*	*To be sipped and swallowed slowly without addition of water.*
Liniments and lotions	*Linimentum and Lotio*	*For external use only.* *Shake the bottle before use.* *Do not apply on broken skin.* (Because it will produce irritation)
Mixtures	*Mistura*	*Shake it well before use.*
Suspensions	*Suspensiō*	*Shake the bottle before use.*
Nasal drops	*Naristillae*	*For nasal use only*
Ointments, Pastes and Paints	*Unguentum, Pasta and pigmentum*	*For external use only.*
Pessaries	*Pessus*	*For vaginal use only*
Suppositories	*Suppositorum*	*For rectal use only.* *Store in a cool place.*

Selection of Containers for Dispensing Medicines

The aim should be to make a clear distinction between preparations that may be taken internally and those intended for external use. The container should also be selected which will best protect the life of the preparation.

Storage conditions and containers for internal or external use:

Preparation	Containers
Cachets	Air tight containers which give adequate physical protection. Containers made of glass, rigid plastics, or extruded aluminum are generally suitable. Use cardboard boxes, which are suitable for short storage periods
Capsules	Airtight containers which give adequate physical protection (Note: Containers made of glass rigid plastics, or extruded aluminum are generally suitable. Suitable internal wadding may be required).
Creams	Wide-mouthed, squat glass jars fitted with plastic screw caps and suitable liners. Certain plastic containers may also be suitable, provided they prevent evaporation of water vapour; plastic containers are unsuitable for those preparations containing plasticizers such as methylsalicylate or phthalate esters.
Draughts	White glass bottles fitted with plastic screw caps with plastic or other impervious liners. Such dose should be packed separately or the exact dose should be made on the label.
Dusting Powders	Cylindrical paper board boxes or plain white glass jars with sprinkler holes on the closure

Contd...

Preparation	Containers
Ear drops	Coloured fluted glass bottles fitted with suitable droppers. Plastic dropper bottles are also suitable provided that the plastic is compatible with the content.
Eye drops	Coloured, fluted glass dropper bottles which are capable of being sterilized by autoclaving. Plastic containers are suitable for some eye-drops provided that the plastic is compatible with the content. (*Note:* The glass must be neutral or soda treated screw-capped dropper bottles and must comply with Indian Pharmacopoeial Standards)
Eye Ointments	Sterile collapsible tubes.
Eye Lotions	Coloured, fluted glass bottles fitted with plastic screw caps with plastic or other impervious liners. Unprotected bulk closures should not be used for eye lotions.
Mouthwashes and gargles	Clear ribbed bottle, glass or plastic, or, amber if contents sensitive to light
Enemas	Coloured fluted glass bottles with plastic screw-caps with plastic or other impervious liners. Disposable flexible plastic containers are suitable for some enemas provided that the plastic is compatible with the content.
Elixirs	Plain white glass bottles fitted with plastic screw-caps with plastic or other impervious liners.
Gargles	White fluted glass bottles fitted with plastic screw-caps with plastic or other impervious liners.
Granules	Airtight containers which give adequate; physical protection containers made of glass, rigid plastics, or extruded aluminum; are generally suitable.
Inhalations	White fluted glass bottles fitted with plastic screw caps with plastic or impervious liners.
Linctuses	Plain white glass bottles fitted with plastic screw caps with plastic or other impervious liners
Liniments	Coloured fluted glass bottles fitted with plastic screw caps with plastic or other impervious liners
Lotions	Coloured fluted glass bottles fitted with plastic screw caps with plastic or other impervious liners.
Lozenges	Airtight containers which give adequate physical protection. Containers made of glass, rigid plastics, or extruded aluminum, are generally suitable.
Mixtures	Plain white non-graduated glass bottles fitted with plastic or other impervious liners
Mouthwashes	White fluted glass bottles fitted with plastic screw caps with plastic or other impervious liners
Nasal drops	Coloured fluted glass bottles with a dropper. Plastic dropper bottles are also suitable, provided that the plastic is compatible with the content.
Ointments	Wide-mouthed, screw-capped, plain squat glass jars or plastic jars metal or plastic flexible tubes with screw caps. Certain plastic containers containing plasticizers such as methyl salicylate ester are not suitable for some ointments

Contd...

Preparation	Containers
Paints	Coloured fluted glass bottles fitted with plastic screw caps with plastic or other impervious liners.
Pastes	Wide-mouthed, screw-capped, plain squat glass or plastic jar metal or; plastic flexible tubes with screw caps.
Pastilles	Airtight containers, which give adequate physical protection, containers made of glass, rigid plastics, or extruded aluminum, are generally suitable
Pessaries	They should be wrapped individually in waxed paper, in metal foil, or in some suitable form of strip packing. They should be dispensed in partitioned boxes or in suitable plastics containers (for 4 g pessaries use 120 g ointment jars).
Powders	Bulk powders should be dispensed in airtight containers, which give adequate physical protection. Containers made of glass, rigid plastics, or extruded Aluminium, are generally suitable. Individually wrapped powders should be dispensed in stout paperboard boxes with bonded plastic membrane, plastic boxes with bonded plastic membrane, plastic boxes or folding paperboard cartons, which give adequate physical protection. Powders containing deliquescent or volatile materials should be double wrapped in greaseproof paper.
Solution Tablets	Airtight containers, which give adequate physical protection. Containers made of glass, rigid plastics, or extruded aluminum, are generally suitable
Spray Solutions	White fluted glass bottles fitted with plastic screw-caps with plastic or other impervious liners
Suppositories	As for pessaries
Tablets	Airtight containers which give adequate physical protection. Containers made of glass, rigid plastics, or extruded aluminum are generally suitable. Foil or strip packed tablets should be packed in suitable paperboard boxes or folding paperboard cartons which give adequate physical protection. Internal wadding may be necessary

Important Conversions, Formulae and Equations

1. Relationship between Celsius degrees ($^\circ$C) and Fahrenheit degrees ($^\circ$F)

    $9(^\circ C) = 5(^\circ F)-160$

2. Density = Weight/Volume or Weight = Density$\times$ Volume

3. Various order of reactions:

Order of Reaction	Equation	Final Concentration	Half-life ($T^{1/2}$)
Zero order	$dc/dt= -k\times c^\circ$	$C=C_o-kt$	$0.5C_o/k$
First order	$dc/dt= -k\times c^1$	$\log C=\log C_o-kt/2.303$	$0.693/k$
Second order	$dc/dt= -k\times c^2$	$1/C=1/ C_o+ kt$	$1/ C_o/k$

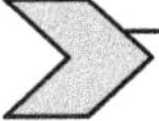

Prescription and its Components

It is defined as a written order by a physician, dentist, veterinarian or a registered medical practitioner to a pharmacist to compound and dispense a specific medication for the patient. It comprises the directions which are provided to the pharmacist about what type of dosage form/preparation (such as powder mixture, syrup, tablet, emulsion or suspension etc.) has to be dispensed by the pharmacist for the patient. Further, it also directs to the pharmacist about the dose of the drug, dosing interval (dosage regimen) and route of administration which has to be followed by the patient. Earlier, prescriptions were written in Latin language so that the prescription content remains unknown to the patients to avoid self medication.

For example: A typical prescription can be depicted as follows:

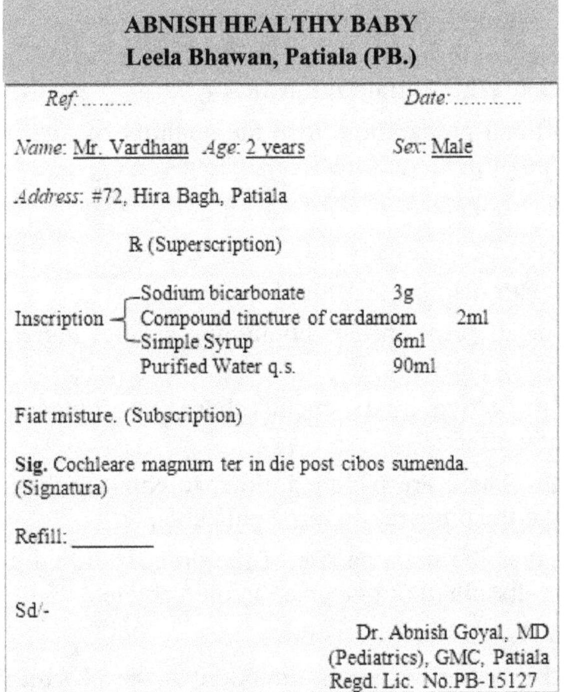

ABNISH HEALTHY BABY
Leela Bhawan, Patiala (PB.)

Ref. ....   Date: ....

Name: Mr. Vardhaan   Age: 2 years   Sex: Male

Address: #72, Hira Bagh, Patiala

R (Superscription)

Inscription
- Sodium bicarbonate   3g
- Compound tincture of cardamom   2ml
- Simple Syrup   6ml
- Purified Water q.s.   90ml

Fiat misture. (Subscription)

Sig. Cochleare magnum ter in die post cibos sumenda. (Signatura)

Refill: _________

Sd/-

Dr. Abnish Goyal, MD
(Pediatrics), GMC, Patiala
Regd. Lic. No.PB-15127

Parts of a Prescription

A typical prescription consists of the following parts:

1. Date

Date on the prescription helps the pharmacists to know when the medicines were last dispensed if the prescription is brought for redispensing of the prescription. In case of habit forming drug the date prevents the misuse of the drug by the patient.

2. Name, age, sex and address of the patient

By name and address the patient and the prescription can be identified. Age and sex of the patient is especially required for child patient to check the prescribed dose.

3. Superscription

It is represented by a Latin symbol ℞, an abbreviation of Latin term '**recipe**' which means '**take thou**' or '**you take**'.

[N.B. In olden days, the symbol was considered to be originated from the sign of Jupiter, the Greek God of healing. This symbol was employed by the ancient in requesting God for the quick recovery of the patient.]

4. Inscription

This is the main part of the prescription. It contains the names and quantities of the prescribed medicaments. The medicament may be official preparation or nonofficial preparation. If is official preparation (i.e. from pharmacopoeia or formulary) then only the name of the preparation is written e.g. Piperazine Citrate Elixir IP.

If it is non-official preparation, then the quantity of each ingredient will be given. The type of preparation will also be given e.g.

Sodium bicarbonate	3 g
Simple Syrup	6 ml
Purified Water q.s.	100 ml

The inscription of prescriptions containing several ingredients are divided into the following parts:

(a) *Base*: The active medicaments those are intended to produce the therapeutic effect.

(b) *Adjuvants*: These are included either to enhance the action of the drug or to make the preparation more palatable.

(c) *Vehicle*: It is the main carrier of the drug. In liquid preparations drugs are either dissolved or dispersed in the vehicle.

5. Subscription

In this part the prescriber gives direction to the pharmacist regarding the dosage form to be prepared and the number of doses to be dispensed.

6. Signatura

It is usually written as '**Sig.**'. The instructions given in the prescription should be written in the label of the container so that the patient can follow them. The instructions may include:

(a) The quantity to be taken (b)   The   frequency   and   timing   of administration of the preparation (c) The route of administration (d) The special instruction (if any).

7. Renewal instructions

The prescriber indicates in every prescription, whether it should be renewed, and if renewed, for how many times. It is very important particularly for habit forming drugs to prevent their misuse.

8. Signature, address and registration number of the prescriber

The prescription must be signed by the prescriber by his / her own hand. His/her address and registration number should be written in the case of dangerous and habit forming drugs.

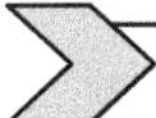 ## Handling of Prescription

The following procedures should be adopted by the pharmacist while handling the prescription for compounding and dispensing:

(i) Receiving

(ii) Reading and checking

(iii) Collecting and weighing the materials

(iv) Compounding, labeling and packaging

(i) Receiving

- The prescription should be received by the pharmacist himself / herself.

- While receiving a prescription from a patient a pharmacist should bot change his/her facial expression that gives an impression to the patient that he/she is confused or surprised after seeing the prescription.

(ii) Reading and checking

- After receiving the prescription, it should be screened behind the counter.

- The prescription is a hospital slip or from a nursing home or from a private practitioner and their authenticity should be checked. The signature of the prescriber and the date of prescription is checked.

- The pharmacist should read all the lines and words of the prescription. He/she must not guess any word. If there is any doubt, the pharmacist should consult with the other pharmacist or the prescriber over telephone.

(iii) Collecting and weighing the material

Before compounding a prescription all the materials required should be collected from the shelves or drawers and kept at the left hand side of the balance. After measuring, each material should be kept on the right hand side of the balance. After compounding the prescription, the materials are replaced back to the shelves / drawers where from they were collected.

While compounding the label of every container of material should be checked thrice in the following manner:

(i) When collected from the shelves/drawers.

(ii) When the materials are measured.

(iii) When the containers are replaced back to the shelves/drawers.

(iv) Compounding, labeling and packaging

- Only one prescription should be compounded at a time.

- Compounding should be done on a clean table.

- All equipment required should be clean and dry.

- The preparation should be prepared according to the direction of the prescriber or as per methods given in pharmacopoeia or formulary are according to established pharmaceutical art of compounding.

Errors in Prescription

1. Dispensing related errors

2. Prescribe related errors

3. Patient related errors

1. Dispensing related errors:

(a) **Abbreviation:** In most of the prescriptions abbreviated terms are used by the prescriber that leads to major errors during interpretation by the pharmacists. E.g. 'SSKI' is the abbreviated term of 'Saturated Solution of Potassium Iodide'. It is preferable to avoid this type of misleading abbreviations.

(b) **Name of the drugs**

Names of some drugs (especially the brand names) either looks or sounds alike. So any error in the name of a drug will lead to major danger to the patient.

e.g. Althrocin – Eltroxin, Acidin – Apidin etc.

(c) **Strength of the preparation**

Drugs are available in the market in various strengths. So a drug must not be dispensed if the strength is not written in the prescription. E.g. Paracetamol tablet 500mg should not be dispensed when no strength is mentioned in the prescription.

(d) **Dosage form of the drug prescribed**

Many drug are available in more than one dosage forms e.g. liquid, tablets, injections or suppositories. The dosage form intended for the patient must be mentioned in the prescription to reduce ambiguity.

(e) Dose

If unusually high or low dose is mentioned in the prescription, then it must be consulted with the prescriber. Some time a sustained release (SR) dosage form is prescribed thrice or more times daily. Actually, SR dosage forms should be given once or twice a day.

(f) Instructions to the patient

Some times the instruction for a certain preparation is either omitted of mentioned partially. The route of administration should be mentioned clearly.

(g) Incompatibilities

It is essential to check that there are no pharmaceutical or therapeutic incompatibilities in the prescription. If more than two medicines are prescribed, then it is the duty of the pharmacist to see whether their interactions will produce any harm to the patient or not. Certain drugs have interactions with food. The pharmacist has to advise the patient about it. e.g., Tetracycline should not be taken with milk or antacid.

2. Prescriber related errors:

(a) Misleading or erroneous references

(b) Ambiguity in handwriting and types documents

(c) Wrong patient errors

(d) Errors in dosage

3. Patient related errors:

(a) Unable to explain symptoms

(b) Hiding co-morbities

(c) Hiding co-medication being taken concomitantly

(d) Self alteration of dose

(e) Self alteration of time of drug administration

(f) Simultaneously consultations with another doctor

Care Required in Dispensing Prescription

Following precautions should be taken while dispensing a prescription.

1. The prescription must be carried with the pharmacist while taking the medicine out of the shelves. It will constantly remind the name and strength of the preparation required.

2. The dispensing balance should always be checked before weighing any ingredient.

3. All the chemicals and stock preparations should be replaced back in to their original positions in the shelf.

4. While pouring or measuring a liquid ingredient care must be taken to prevent surplus liquid running down of the bottle and staining the label.

5. Care should be taken to keep the balance clean after each measurement. The powders should be transferred by a clean spatula.

6. Liquid preparations for external use should be supplied in a fluted bottle and the label must display FOR EXTERNAL USE ONLY in red ink.

7. Before handing over the medicine to the patient, again the preparation should be checked that the correct preparation, in the correct strength, has been supplied and the correct direction has been stated on the label.

Labeling of Dispensed Medicines

After dispensing the medicine in a container, a label is attached by adhesive. The label on the dispensed medicines should provide the following information: –

1. **Name of the preparation**

   When the prescriber mentions the name in the prescription the same name must be displayed on the label.

   e.g.   PIPERAZINE CITRATE ELIXIR IP

   If it is a non-official preparation, then the name of the dosage form should be given on the label.

   e.g.   THE MIXTURE, THE EMULSION, THE DUSTING POWDER

2. **The strength of the medicine**

   The strength of the active ingredient in the preparation must be displayed if it is intended for internal (oral) purpose.

   The amount in each unit of dose should be mentioned.

   e.g. In case of oral liquids "Each 5ml contains 250 mg"

   e.g. In case of tablet "Each tablet contains 500 mg".

   The values must be written in whole numbers and if decimal is not avoidable then a zero is placed before the decimal point. E.g. instead of 0.1 g it should be 100 mg, and instead of .5% it should be 0.5%.

   In case of an official preparation the strength is not required to be given, because the name with reference to the pharmacopoeia is sufficient.

   e.g. Chloramphenicol Oral Suspension I.P.

3. **The quantity supplied in the container**

   The total quantity of the product dispensed in the container should be indicated on the label. E.g. 50 ml, 4tabs etc.

4. **Storage conditions and shelf life (expiry date) of the product**

   (a) *Temperature:* Many preparations are required to be kept below 15^{0}C. In these cases the label should indicate KEEP IN A COOL PLACE.

Suppositories and pessaries melts at 37^0C so the label should indicate KEEP IN A COOL PLACE.

Insulin injections should be stored at 2 to 8^0C so the label should indicate KEEP IN REFRIGERATOR.

(b) *Humidity*: Powders, tablets and capsules should be stored in an air-tight container. The label should indicate KEEP THE BOTTLE TIGHTLY CLOSED.

(c) *Light*: Drugs those degrade in presence of light should be stored in dark place. The label should indicate KEEP IN A DARK PLACE.

5. Instructions to the patient

(a) *Directions*

The directions are normally written by the prescriber. These include

(i)   the quantity to be taken

(ii) the frequency or timing of administration

(iii) the route of administration

(iv) or the method of use

The phrases used are generally '*to be taken*', '*to be given*', or '*to be used*'.

e.g. One tablet to be taken thrice daily after meal.

(b) *Warning label*:

For external use only.	In case of external preparations like ointment, pastes, dusting powders etc.
Drowsiness warning.	*Warning*: May cause drowsiness. Do not drive or operate machinery or car.
Potential interactions with food or drink	(i) Drugs in which absorption improves if taken before food: *Warning*: To be taken an hour before meal or in empty stomach. (ii) Drugs causing gastrointestinal irritation *Warning*: To be taken with or after meal. (iii) In case of metronidazole *Warning*: Avoid alcoholic drink.
Interactions with other medicine	Tetracycline complexes with calcium, iron, magnesium and inhibits its absorption, *Warning*: Do not take milk, iron preparation or antacids with this medicine.
Special methods of administration	(i) The drug formulation that is required to be dissolved in the mouth *Warning*: To be sucked or chewed. (ii) Oral powders or granules are required to be dissolved in water *Warning*: To be dissolved in water before taking. (iii) Drugs causing gastro-intestinal irritation *Warning: To be taken with plenty of water.*

Contd...

Cautions	(i) Preparation that may produce photosensitization *Warning*: Avoid exposure of skin to direct sunlight. (ii) The preparation that may produce unusual effect. *Warning*: The preparation may color the urine or stool. (iii) In case of inflammable preparation *Warning*: Keep away from naked flame.

Common Latin Terms Used in Prescriptions

Latin term	Abbreviation	English meaning
Auristillae	Auristill.	Ear drops
Charta	Chart	Powder
Collutorium	Collut.	Mouthwash
Collyrium	Collyr.	Eye lotion
Cremor	Crem.	Cream
Emulsio	Emul.	Emulsion
Gargarisma	Garg.	Galgle
Guttae	Gtt.	Drops
Guttur pigmentum	Gtt. Pigm.	Drops
Haustus	Ht	Draught
Inhalatio	Inhal.	Inhalation
Insufflatio	Insuff	Insufflation
Linimentum	Lin.	Liniment
Liquor	Liq.	Solution
Lotio	Lot.	Lotion
Mistura	Mist.	Mixture
Oculus guttae	Ocul. Gtt.	Eye drops
Oculentum	Oculent.	Eye ointment
Pulvis	Pulv.	Powder
Pulvis consperus	Pulv. Consper	Dusting powder
Sternutamentum	Sternut	Snuff
Trochiscus	Troch.	Lozenge
Unguentum	Ung.	Ointment
Applicandus	Applicand.	To be applied
Ad usum externum	Ad. Us. Enter.	For eternal use
Capiendus	Capiend.	To be taken
Consperge	Consper.	Dust, sprinkle
Dolore urgente	Dol. Urg.	When pain is severe
Infricandus	Infricand	To be rubbed
Quantum libitum	q. lib.	As much as you wish

Contd...

Latin term	Abbreviation	English meaning
Quantum sufficiat	q.s.	As much as is sufficient
Sine	s	Without
Pro usu externo	Pro. Us. Exter.	For external use
Ut dictum	Ut. Dict.	As directed
More dicto	m.d.	As directed
Prorenata	p.r.n.	Occcasionally
Si opus sit	s.o.s	Whenever necessary or required
Statim	Stat.	Immediately
Semel in die	Sem in die	Once a day
Bis in die	b.i.d.	Twice a day
Ter in die	t.i.d.	Thrice a day
Quarter in die	q.i.d.	Four times a day
Sexies in die	Se i. d.	Six times a day
Bis terve die	b.t.i.d.	Two or three times a day
Ter quaterve die	t.q.d.	Three or four times a day
Quaque hora	qq.h.	Every hour
Singulis hora	Sing. Hor.	Every one hour
Cibos (cibum)	C	Meal
Hora decubitus	h.d.	At bed time
Quoties opus sit	Quot.o.s.	As often as necessary
Primo mane	Prim. M.	Early in the morning
Prima luce	Prim. Luc.	Early in the morning
Mane	M	In the morning
Omni mane	o. m.	Every morning
Omni nocte	o.n.	Every night
Inter nocte	Inter noct.	During the night
Jentaculum	Jentac.	Breakfast
Nocte manaque	n. m.	Night and morning
Omni quarta hora	o.q.h.	Every four hour
Quaaue secunda hora	qq. sec. h.	Every alternate hour
Alternis horis	Alt. hor.	Every two hours
Tertiis horis	Tert. Hor.	Every three hours
Ante cibos	a.c.	Before meals
Post		After
Post cibos	p. c.	After meals
Inter cibos	i.c.	Between meals
Cochleare amplum	Coch. Amp.	One tablespoonful
Cochleare magnum	Coch. Mag.	One tablespoonful
Cochleare maximum	Coch. Max.	One tablespoonful
Cochleare parvem	Coch. Parv.	One tea spoonful
Cochleare infans	Coch. Inf.	One tea spoonful
Cochleare minimum	Coch. Min.	One tea spoonful
Cochleare medium	Coch. Med.	One desertspoonful

Contd...

Latin term	Abbreviation	English meaning
Ex lacte	e. lact.	With milk
E aqua	Ex. Aq.	With water
Misce	m.	Mix
Partes aequalis	p.a.	Equal parts
Ad	Ad.	To, upto
Ana	Aa	F each
Ante	A	Before
Pro dosi		As a dose

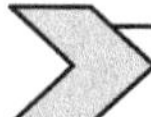

Posology

'Posology' refers to calculation of doses for children.

Factors affecting posology: The factors which affect the posology are listed as hereunder:

1. **Age**: Human beings can be categorized into the following age groups:

Neonate	Up to 1 month from birth
Infant	Up to 1 year age
Child in between	*1 to 4 years*
Child in between	*5 to 12 years*
Adult	Up to 60 years from 16 years
Geriatric (elderly) patients	>60 years

In children the enzyme systems in the liver and renal excretion remain less developed. So all the dose should be less than that of an adult. In elderly patients the renal functions decline. Metabolism rate in the liver also decreases. Drug absorption from the intestine becomes slower in elderly patients. So in geriatric patients the dose is less and should be judiciously administered.

2. **Sex**: Special care should be taken while administering any drug to a woman during menstruation, pregnancy and lactation. Strong purgatives should not be given in menstruation and pregnancy. Antimalarials, ergot alkaloids should not be taken during pregnancy to avoid deformation of foetus. Antihistaminic and sedative drugs are not taken during breast feeding because these drugs are secreted in the milk and the child may be affected by consuming them.

3. **Body size**: It influences the concentration of drug in the body. The average adult dose is calculated for a person with 70 kg body weight (BW). For exceptionally obese (fat) or lean (thin) patient the dose may be calculated on body weight basis.

$$\text{Individual dose} = \frac{\text{Body Weight (kg)}}{70} \times \text{Average adult dose}$$

Another method of dose calculation is according to the *body surface area* (BSA). This method is more accurate than the body weight method.

$$\text{Individual dose} = \frac{\text{Body surface area (m}^2)}{1.7} \times \text{Average adult dose}$$

The body surface area (BSA) of an individual can be obtained from the following formula:

$$\text{BSA (m}^2) = \text{BW(kg)}^{0.425} \times \text{Height (cm)}^{0.725} \times 0.007184$$

4. **Route of administration**

   In case of intravenous injection, the total drug reach immediately to the systemic circulation hence the dose is less in i.v. injection than through oral route or any other route.

5. **Time of administration**

   The drugs are most quickly absorbed from empty stomach. The presence of food in the stomach delays the absorption of drugs. Hence a potent drug is given before meal. Drug irritant to the stomach is given after meal so that the drug is diluted with food and thus produces less irritation.

6. **Environmental factors**

   Stimulant types of drug are taken at day time and sedative types of drugs are taken at night. So the dose of a sedative required in day time will be much higher than at night.

7. **Psychological state**

   Psychological state of mind can affect the response of a drug, e.g. a nervous and anxious patient requires more general anaesthetics. *Placebo* is an inert substance that does not contain any drug. Commonly used placebos are *lactose tablets and distilled water injections*. Some time patients often get some psychological effects from this *placebo*. Placebos are more often used in clinical trials of drugs.

8. **Pathological states (i.e. Presence of disease)**

   Several diseases may affect the dose of drugs:

   In *gastrointestinal disease* like *achlorhydria* (reduced secretion of HCl acid in the stomach) the absorption of aspirin decreases.

   In *liver disease* (like liver cirrhosis) metabolism of some drugs (like morphine, pentobarbitone etc.) decreases.

   In *kidney diseases* excretion of drugs (like aminoglycosides, digoxin, phenobarbitone) is reduced, so less dose of the drugs should be administered.

9. Accumulation

Any drug will accumulate in the body if the rate of absorption is more than the rate of elimination. Slowly eliminated drugs are often accumulated in the body and often causes toxicity e.g. prolonged use of chloroquin causes damage to retina.

10. Drug interactions

Simultaneous administration of two drugs may result in same or increased or decrease effects.

Drug administration with dose	Pharmacological effect
Drug A	Effect A
Drug B	Effect B
Drug A + Drug B	Effect AB

Relationship	Name of the effect	Examples
Effect AB = Effect A + Effect B	Additive effect	Aspirin + Paracetamol
Effect AB > Effect A + Effect B	Synergistic (or potentiation)	Sulfamethaxazole + Trimethoprim
Effect AB < Effect A + Effect B	Antagonism	Histamine + Adrenaline

11. Idiosyncrasy

This an exceptional response to a drug in few individual patients. For example, in some patients, aspirin may cause asthma, penicillin causes irritating rashes on the skin etc.

12. Genetic diseases

Some patients may have genetic defects. They lack some enzymes. In those cases some drugs are contraindicated.

e.g. Patients lacking *Glucose-6-phosphate dehydrogenase* enzyme should not be given *primaquine* (an antimalarial drug) because it will cause hemolysis.

13. Tolerance

Some time higher dose of a drug is required to produce a given response (*previously less dose was required*).

Natural Tolerance: Some races are inherently less sensitive to some drugs, e.g. rabbits and black race (Africans) are more tolerant to atropine.

Acquired Tolerance: By repeated use of a drug in an individual for a long time require larger dose to produce the same effect that was obtained with normal dose previously.

Cross tolerance: It is the development of tolerance to pharmacologically related drugs e.g. alcoholics are relatively more tolerant to sedative drugs.

Tachyphylaxis: (*Tachy* = fast, *phylaxis* = protection) is rapid development of tolerance. When a dose of a drug is repeated in quick succession a reduction in response occurs – this is called *tachyphylaxis*. This is usually seen in ephedrine, nicotine.

Drug resistance: It refers to tolerance of microorganisms to inhibitory action of antimicrobials e.g. *Staphylococci* to penicillin.

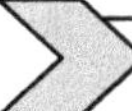 ## Pediatric Dose Calculations

Various Formulas for Calculation of Doses

Based on Age

1. Young's Formula

$$\text{Dose of Child} = \frac{\text{Age of child (years)}}{\text{Age of child (years)} + 12} \times \text{Adult dose}$$

2. Dilling's Formula

$$\text{Dose of Child} = \frac{\text{Age of child (years)}}{20} \times \text{Adult dose}$$

3. Cowling's Formula

$$\text{Dose of Child} = \frac{\text{Age of child (years)} + 1}{24} \times \text{Adult dose}$$

4. Fried's Formula

$$\text{Dose of Child} = \frac{\text{Age of child (months)}}{150} \times \text{Adult dose}$$

5. Bastedo's Formula

$$\text{Dose of Child} = \frac{\text{Age of child (years)} + 3}{30} \times \text{Adult dose}$$

Based on Body Weight

Clark's Formula

$$\text{Dose of Child} = \frac{\text{Weight of child (pounds)}}{150 \text{ (pounds)}} \times \text{Adult dose}$$

$$\text{Dose of Child} = \frac{\text{Weight of child (kilograms)}}{70} \times \text{Adult dose}$$

Based on Body Surface Area Method

Nomogram based on Dubois method:

$$BSA\ (m^2) = \frac{(Height)cm \times Weight(kg)^{1/2}}{60}$$

Catzel's Rule

$$Dose\ of\ Child = \frac{Body\ surface\ area\ of\ child}{Body\ surface\ area\ of\ adult\ (1.73M^2)} \times Adult\ dose$$

Mosteller's Rule: A most accurate method commonly used in oncology settings.

$$BSA\ (M^2) = \sqrt{\frac{ht(cm) \times wt(kg)}{3600}}$$

Calculation of Child Doses

Age	Weight (kg)	Height (cm)	BSA (m²)	Fraction of adult dose		
				Young's rule	Clark's Rule	BSA method
Birth	3.5	50.5	0.21	–	0.05	0.12
3 mos	5.7	59.9	0.29	0.02	0.08	0.17
6 mos	7.5	65.8	0.35	0.04	0.11	0.20
1 yr	9.9	74.7	0.44	0.08	0.15	0.25
2 yrs	12.5	86.9	0.54	0.14	0.18	0.31
3 yrs	14.5	96.0	0.61	0.20	0.21	0.35
4 yrs	16.5	103.4	0.68	0.25	0.24	0.39
5 yrs	19.1	110.5	0.76	0.29	0.28	0.44
6 yrs	21.5	116.8	0.84	0.33	0.32	0.49
7 yrs	24.2	123.2	0.91	0.37	0.35	0.53
8 yrs	26.9	129.0	0.98	0.40	0.39	0.57
9 yrs	29.5	134.1	1.04	0.43	0.43	0.60
10 yrs	32.3	139.4	1.12	0.45	0.47	0.65
11 yrs	35.5	144.5	1.20	0.48	0.52	0.69
12 yrs	39.1	150.9	1.28	0.60	0.57	0.74

Practice Example: What will be the dose for a child of 6 years if the adult dose is 500 mg.

Reducing and enlarging formulae (recipe)

In order to prepare any pharmaceutical product, it is necessary to make it from a *master formula* or *official formula*. This master formula may be scaled down or scaled up depending on the requirement.

Rules for conversion of the formula

1. Determine the total weight or volume of the whole preparation.

2. Calculate the ratio of $\dfrac{\text{amount to be prepared}}{\text{total amount of the preparation}}$.

This is called *conversion factor*.

3. Multiply the *conversion factor* with the quantity of each ingredient. The unit should be unchanged.

Example of reducing the recipe

The master formula: Give the working formula for 100 ml preparation.

Ingredient	Quantity required
Drug X	120 g
Sucrose	480 g
Purified water q.s.	1000 ml

The total volume of the preparation is 1000 ml. Required volume of the preparation is 100 ml.

So the conversion factor is $\dfrac{100}{1000} = 0.1$

The reduced formula

Ingredient	Quantity required for 1000 ml	Conversion factor	Quantity required for 100 ml
Drug X	120 g		12.0 g
Sucrose	480 g	100/1000 = 0.1	48.0 g
Purified water q.s.	1000 ml		100 ml

Example of enlarging the recipe

The master formula: Give the working formula for 2.5 L

Ingredient	Quantity required
Liquid P	35 ml
Solid A	9 g
Liquid R	2.5 ml
Liquid S	20 ml
Purified water q.s.	100 ml

Total volume of the preparation is 100 ml. Required volume of the preparation is 2.5 L i.e. 2500 ml.

So the conversion factor is $\dfrac{2500}{100} = 25$

The enlarged formula

Ingredient	Quantity required for 1000 ml	Conversion factor	Quantity required for 100 ml
Liquid P	35 ml		875 ml
Solid A	9 g	2500/100 = 25	225 g
Liquid R	2.5 ml		62.5 ml
Liquid S	20 ml		500 ml
Purified water q.s.	100 ml		2500 ml

Exercise: Calculate the amount of ingredients required for preparing 30g of ointment.

Ingredient	Quantity required for 1000 g	Conversion factor	Quantity required for 30 g
Wool fat	50 g		1.5 g
Hard Paraffin	50 g	30/1000 = 0.03	1.5 g
Cetostearyl alcohol	50 g		1.5 g
White soft paraffin	850 g		25.5 g
	Total = 1000 g		

Typical Label for a Formulation

CALAMINE LOTION I.P. 40 ml	
INGREDIENTS	
Calamine	06.0 g
Zinc Oxide	02.0 g
Bentonite	01.2 g
Sodium Citrate	00.2 g
Liquefied Phenol	00.2 ml
Glycerin	02.0 ml
Rose Water q.s.	40.0 ml

MANUFACTURED BY: ABC Pharmaceuticals

MFG. DATE:

EXP. DATE:

USE: Use on skin rashes, minor burns and infections

DOSE:

STORAGE: Keep in cool place

FOR EXTERNAL USE ONLY

Dispensed By:

Adult Doses of Few Important Drugs

Category	Drug	Dose	Dosage regimen
ANALGESICS	Metamizole Sodium	500 mg	3-4 times a day
	Aspirin(Dispersible)	350 mg	3 times a day
	Ibuprofen	400 mg	4 times a day
	Rofecoxib	12.5/25/50 mg	Once Daily
	Celecoxib	50/100/200 mg	Twice Daily
	Etoricoxib	30/60/90/120 mg	Once Daily
ANTI PYRETICS	Paracetamol	500 mg	Three times daily
	Nimesulide	100 mg	2 times a day
ANTIBIOTICS	Amoxicillin	500 mg	Every 8 to 12 h
	Ciprofloxacin	500 mg	2 times a day
	Azithromycin	250/500 mg	Once daily
	Roxithromycin	200/400 mg	Twice daily
	Ofloxacin	200/400 mg	Twice daily
ANTIHYPERTENSIVES	Clonidine	100/150/300 μg	1 or 2 times a day as prescribed
	Atenolol	50 mg	
	Lisinopril	7.5/15 mg	Once daily
	Amlodipine	10/20 mg	Once daily
	Valsartan	40/80/120 mg	Once daily
	Candesartan	4/8/16/32 mg	Twice daily
	Telmisartan	20/40/80 mg	Once daily
	Olmesartan	5/20/40 mg	Once daily
			Once daily
ANTI DIABETICS	Glipizide	5 mg	1 or 2 times a day as prescribed
	Metformin	500/1000 mg	Twice daily
	Canagliflozin	100 mg	Once daily
ANTI VIRALS	Acyclovir	400 mg	Thrice daily (10 days)
	Rimantidine	100 mg	Once daily
	Zidovudine(HIV)	300 mg	Twice daily
ANTI HISTAMINIC	Cetirizine	10 mg tab	Once daily
	Levoctirizine	5 mg tab	Once daily
	Diphenhydramine	25/50 mg	Once daily
	Fexofinadine	60/180 mg	Once daily
ANTI AMOEBIC	Metronidazole	700 mg	Thrice daily for 5-7 days
	Tinidazole	2 g	Once daily for 3-6 days
	Paromomycin	500 mg	Thrice daily for 7 days
	Ornidazole	500-1000 mg	Once /Twice Daily

Contd...

Category	Drug	Dose	Dosage regimen
ANTI ASTHEMATICS	Noscapine	1.4 mg/ml syrup	Twice daily
	Salbutamol	2/4 mg	Once daily
	Montelukast	10 mg	Once daily
	Zafirlukast	10/20 mg	20 mg (Twice daily)
STEROIDAL DRUGS	Prednisolone		5-60 mg/day
	Betamethasone		0.5-5 mg /day
	Fludrocortisone		50-200 µg daily
ANTI MIGRAINE	Sumatriptan	50,100 mg tab	Once daily
	Ergotamine	2 mg	Once daily
	Rizatriptan	5/10 mg	Once daily
ANTI LIPIDEMIC	Atorvastatin	10/20/40/80 mg	Once daily
	Fluvastatin	20/40/80 mg	Once daily

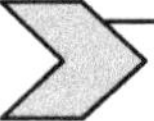

Pharmaceutical Calculations

Weights and measures:

There are two systems of weights and measurements- Imperial and Metric system. The imperial system is traditional system of weight and measures categorized into systems- Avoirdupois and Apothecaries (also known as Troy System). In Avoidupois system, pound (lb) is the standard unit of weight and all measures of mass is derived from it whereas in Apothecaries system, grain is the standard unit of weight and all measures of mass is derived from it.

Measurements of weights in imperial system

Weight is a measure of the gravitational force acting on a body and is directly proportional to its mass.

(a) Avoirdupois system

In this system **pound (lb)** is taken as the standard of weight (mass).

1 pound avoir (lb)	= 16 oz avoir	**oz** is pronounced as *ounce.*
1 pound avoir (lb)	= 7000 grains (gr)	

(b) Apothecary or Troy system

In this system **grain (gr)** is taken as the standard of weight (mass).

1 pound apoth (lb)	= 12 ounces (℥)	
1 ounce (℥)	= 8 drachms (ʒ)	1 pound apoth (lb) = 5760 grains (gr)
1 drachm (ʒ)	= 3 scruples (℈)	
1 scruple (℈)	= 20 grains (gr)	

In summary, the conversion of various units between Avoirdupois and Apothecaries systems has been listed hereunder:

Apothecaries system	Avoidupois system
1 Lb	16 oz or 7000 gr
1oz	437.5 gr
20 grains (gr)	1 scruple
60 grains	1 drachm
480 grains	1 ounce (apothe)
12 ounces	1 pound (apothe)
5760 grains	1 pound (apothe)

Weights in metric system: This system is used in Indian pharmacopoeia (I.P) for measurements of weights and volume and was implemented in India w.e.f. 01.04.1964 in pharmacy profession. A kilogram is the standard unit of weight and all measures of mass are derived from it.

Units	Abbreviated symbols	Equivalent to grams (g)
1 microgram	µg or mcg	0.000,001
1 milligram	Mg	0.001
1 centigram	Cg	0.01
1 decigram	Dg	0.1
1 gram	G	1.0
1 dekagram	Dag	10.0
1 hectogram	Hg	100.0
1 kilogram	Kg	1000.0

Linear measurements in metric system:

Units	Abbreviated symbols	Equivalent to meter(m)
1 inch	In	0.0254
1 nanometer	Nm	1e-9
1 A (angstrom unit)	Å	1e-10
1 micrometer	µm	1e-6
1 millimeter	Mm	0.001
1 centimeter	Cm	0.01
1 decimeter	Dm	0.1
1 meter	M	1.0
1 dekameter	Dam	10
1 hectometer	Hm	100
1 kilometer	Km	1000.0

Measurements of Volumes in Imperical System

1 gallon (c)	= 4 quarts = 160 fl. ounces = 8 pints
1 quart	= 2 pint (o)= 40 fl. ounces
1 pint (o)	= 20 fluid ounce
1 fluid ounce	= 8 fluid drachm= 480 minims
1 fluid drachm	= 3 fluid scruple
1 fluid scruple	= 20 minims

Example:

Convert (i) *quart to minim*

$$1 \text{ quart} = 2 \text{ pint}$$

$$= 2 \times (20 \text{ fluid ounce})$$

$$= 2 \times 20 \times (8 \text{ fluid drachm})$$

$$= 2 \times 20 \times 8 \times (3 \text{ fluid scruple})$$

$$= 2 \times 20 \times 8 \times 3 \times (20 \text{ minims})$$

$$= 19200 \text{ minims}$$

(ii) pint to fluid ounce, (iii) fluid ounce to minim, fluid drachm = minim

Measurements of volumes in metric system

Units	Abbreviated symbols	Equivalent to litres (L)
1 microlitre	μL	0.000,001
1 millilitre	mL	0.001
1 centilitre	cL	0.01
1 decilitre	dL	0.1
1 litre	L	1.0
1 dekalitre	daL	10.0
1 hectolitre	hL	100.0
1 kilolitre	kL	1000.0

Percentage Calculations

Percentages are also commonly used to express the strength of solutions. Usually these solutions are not intended for the oral route of administration. As a percentage this can have four different meanings and in order to make clear the intention the following terms are used:

➤ **% w/w percentage weight in weight.** This expresses the amount in grams of solute in 100 g of product.

➤ **% w/v percentage weight in volume.** This expresses the amount in grams of solute in 100 ml of product.

➤ **% v/v percentage volume in volume.** This expresses the number of millilitres of solute in 100 ml of product.

➤ **% v/w percentage volume in weight.** This expresses the number of millilitres of solute in 100 g of product.

The strength of solutions of solids in liquids is usually expressed as % w/v, whereas that of liquids in liquids is expressed as % v/v. When the type of percentage is not specified by convention the above rule will apply. For example, % solid in liquid is interpreted as % w/v.

Weight in volume (w/v)

In this case the general formula for 1% (w/v) is:

		The formula is actually:	
Solute	1part by weight	Solute	1 g
Solvent upto	100 parts by volume	Solvent upto	100 ml

Exercise 1: Calculate the quantity of sodium chloride required for 500ml of 0.9% solution.

Ans: 0.9%w/v solution of sodium chloride $= \dfrac{0.9\text{g Sodium chloride}}{100\text{ml solution}}$

So 500ml solution will contain

$$\frac{0.9\text{g Sodium chloride}}{100\text{ml solution}} \times 500\text{ml} = \frac{0.9\text{g} \times 500\text{ml}}{100\text{ml}} = \frac{0.9 \times 500}{100}\,\text{g} = 4.5\,\text{g sodium chloride}$$

Exercise 2: Send 100ml of a solution of potassium permanganate of which one part diluted with seven parts of water makes a 1 in 8000 solutions.

Ans.   The planning of calculation is as follows:

Original solution	*Dilution of the solution*	*Final solution* after dilution
Solution of potassium permanganate, x % w/v, 100ml	Solution, x % w/v = 1ml Water = 7ml Volume of solution = 8ml	Potassium permanganate = 1g Volume of solution= 8000ml

So, we have to calculate x. Let us start from final solution.

Concentration of $KMnO_4$ is the final solution $= \dfrac{1\text{g}}{8000\text{ml}} \times 100\text{ml}\,\%(w/v) =$

0.0125 %w/v

Method-1

Let us restructure the problem:

1 ml of x% w/v solution is diluted to a solution of 0.0125%w/v and the final volume is 8ml.

$V1 = 1ml$ $V2 = 8ml$

$S1 = x\%w/v$ $S2 = 0.0125\%w/v$

$V1 \times S1 = V2 \times S2$

Or,   1ml x X% = 8ml x 0.0125%

Or, $X\% = \dfrac{8ml \times 0.0125\%}{1ml}$

Or,   X% = 0.1%

Or,   X = 0.1

Method-2

Concentration of initial solution = ?

Concentration of diluted solution = 0.0125% (w/v)

1 ml diluted to 8ml, so dilution factor = 8, i.e. the solution is diluted 8 times

Concentration of initial solution = Concentration of diluted solution × 8 = 0.0125% w/v × 8 = 0.1%w/v

Ans. A 0.1%w/v potassium permanganate solution is to be prepared.

Exercise 3: Send 250ml of 4 percent potassium permanganate solution and label with directions for preparing 1 liter quantities of a 1 in 2500 solution.

Ans. The planning of calculation is as follows:

Original solution	Dilution of the solution	*Final solution* after dilution
Solution of potassium permanganate, 4 % w/v, 250ml	Solution, 4 % w/v = 1ml Water = ?	Potassium permanganate = 1g Volume of solution = 2500ml

Now do it yourself. Do it by Method-2.

Ans: 100 times dilution i.e. 1 ml is diluted with 99ml water to obtain 100ml solution.

Weight in weight (w/w)

In this case the general formula for 1%(w/w) is:

		The formula is actually:	
Solute	1part by weight	Solute	1 g
Solvent upto	100 parts by weight	Solvent up to	100 g

Problem: Prepare 100ml Phenol Glycerin BPC. It contains 16%w/w phenol in glycerol. Sp.gr. of glycerol = 1.26

Let us assume that phenol is not increasing the volume of the solution.

So the final solution: Volume = 100ml

Volume of glycerol = 100ml

Weight of glycerol = 100ml × 1.26 g/ml = 100 × 1.26 g = 126g

So the working formula will be:

Ingredient	Quantity for 100g	Quantity required for 100ml
Glycerol	84g	126g
Phenol	16g	$\dfrac{16g}{84g} \times 126g = \quad 24g$

Volume in volume (v/v)

In this case the general formula for 1%(w/w) is:

		The formula is actually:	
Solute	1part by volume	Solute	1 ml
Solvent upto	100 parts by volume	Solvent upto	100 ml

Problem: Prepare 600ml of 60%v/v alcohol from 95% v/v alcohol.

In this problem: $V1 = ?$ $S1 = 95\%$ $V2 = 600ml$ $S2 = 60\%$

$$V1 \times S1 = V2 \times S2 \quad \text{or, } V1 = \frac{V2 \times S2}{S1} = \frac{600ml \times 60\%}{95\%} = 379ml$$

Ans: 379 ml of 95% alcohol is diluted to 600ml to obtain 60% alcohol.

Alligation Method

This method is used to calculate the exact proportions in which substances of different strength or concentration are added to yield a mixture of desired strength or concentration.

Rules 1- The desired percent (%) or concentration is placed in central position.

Rule 2-The lower percent (%) or concentration is placed on the left side below the center.

Rule 3- The higher percent (%) or concentration is placed on the left side above the center.

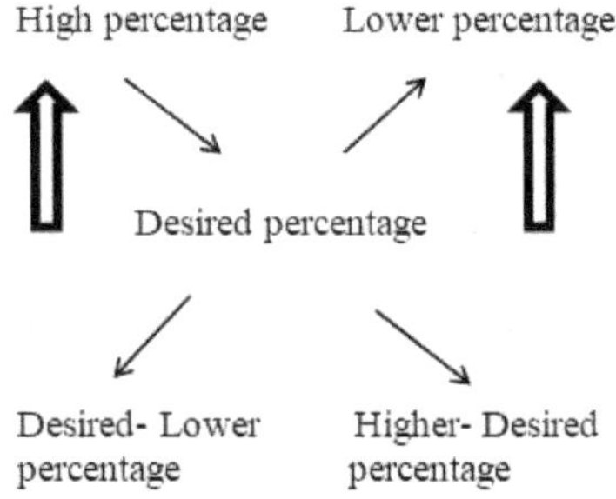

Example: In what proportion must a preparation containing 13% of drug be mixed with one 7% of drug to produce a mixture of 15% desired strength?

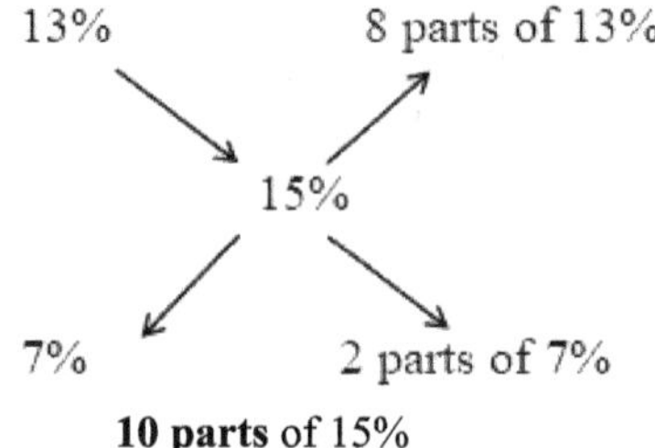

10 parts of 15%

The desired proportion is obtained by subtracting the 7% from 13% and is placed opposite the 13% on the right side and that obtained by subtracting the 15% from 13% is placed opposite the 7% figure on the right side.

Hence, 8 parts of 13% drug mixed with 2 parts of 7% drug shall produce drug mixture of desired strength.

Example: How many grams of 2.5% hydrocortisone cream should be mixed with 360gm of 0.25% cream to make a 1% hydrocortisone cream?

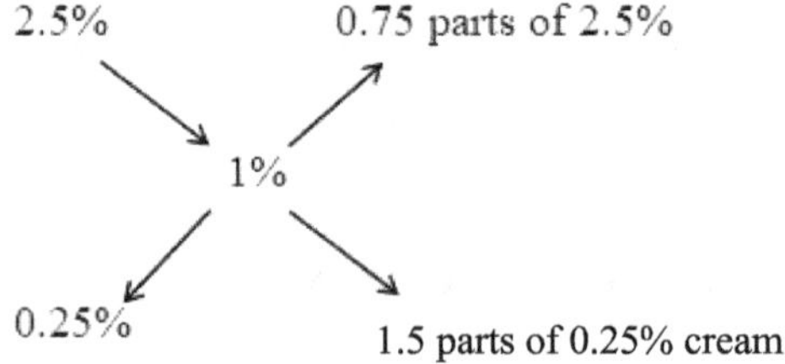

For 2gm of 0.25% = 1gm of 2.5% cream is used

Therefore, for 360gm of 0.25% = 180gm of 2.5% cream is used.

Example: How many grams of coal tar should be added to 3200gm of 5% coal tar ointment to prepare an ointment containing 20% coal tar?

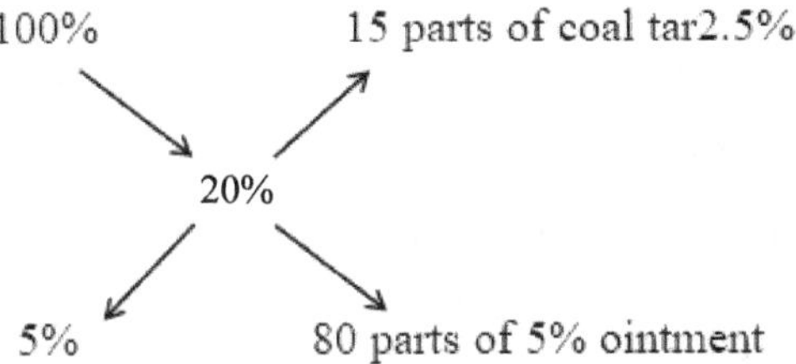

For 16gm of 5% ointment = 3gm of 100% coal tar is needed

Therefore, for 3200gm of 5% ointment $= \dfrac{3200 \times 3}{16} = 600$gm of coal tar is needed.

Example: How many ml of 50% (w/v) dextrose solution and how many ml of 5% (w/v) dextrose solution are required to prepare 4500ml of a 10% (w/v) solution.

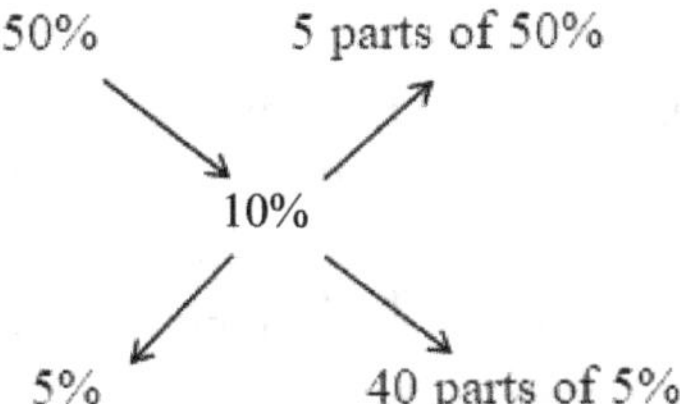

For 9 parts = 1 part of 50% is needed

Therefore, for 4500ml $= \dfrac{4500 \times 1}{9} = 500$ml of 50% solution is required.

For 9 parts = 8 part of 5% solution is needed

Therefore, for 4500ml $= \dfrac{4500 \times 8}{9}$ 4500 x 8 = 4000ml of 5% solution is required.

Millimolar calculations

The strength of active ingredient within a pharmaceutical preparation can be expressed as the number of millimoles per unit volume or mass of product. The mole is the unit of amount of substance and there are 1000 millimoles in a mole.

To calculate the number of millimoles of an ingredient in a medicinal product, you will firstly need to know the molecular weight of the ingredient. The number of moles of ingredient is the mass of ingredient divided by the molecular mass:

$$\text{Number of moles} = \frac{\text{Mass in grams}}{\text{Molecular Mass}}$$

For example, the molecular weight quoted for Sodium Chloride BP is 58.44. Therefore a molar solution of Sodium Chloride BP would contain 58.44 g of Sodium Chloride BP in a litre.

Example: Prepare 100 ml of Sodium Chloride BP solution containing 1.5 mmol per ml.

Answer:

1 ml contains 1.5 mmol or 100 ml contains 150 mmol

1 mole (1000 mmol) of Sodium Chloride BP weighs = 58.44 g

1 mmol of Sodium Chloride BP weighs =58.44/1000 g

150 mmol of Sodium Chloride BP weighs =58.44/1000 g × 150 g = **8.766 g**

Proof Spirits:

In the United States Pharmacopoeia, all alcohol concentrations are expressed as volume-in-volume, based on the quantity of absolute alcohol present, as determined at 15.56 °C. Proof spirit was official in B.P. 1885. London Proof spirit means that mixture of ethyl alcohol and water which weighs exactly 12/13th part of an equal volume of distilled water at 51°F.

As per Indian standards, strength of alcohol is measured in proof degrees. Proof spirit has a sp. gr. of 091976 at 15.5 °C and contains 57.1% v/v of ethyl alcohol is said to be 100 volume of proof spirit or 100° Proof. Proof spirit is therefore an aqueous solution containing 57.1% v/v of absolute alcohol.

In India the rates of excise duty are prescribed in terms of rupees per litre of proof alcohol. Thus, any %v/v of alcohol can be converted into proof strength and vice versa using the following method.

1. Multiply the percent strength of alcohol by 1.753 and deduct 100 from the product.

2. If the result is positive, it is termed as over proof (°O/P) means strength of alcohol above the proof strength.

3. If the result is negative, it is termed as under proof (°U/P) means strength of alcohol below proof strength.

Therefore, 25 (°U/P) mean that 100 volume of such alcohol are equivalent to 100-25 = 75 volume of proof sprit. 35 (°O/P) mean that 100 volume of such alcohol are equivalent to $100 + 35 = 135$ volume of proof spirit.

In summary,

Proof spirit is that mixture of alcohol and water, which at 51^0F weighs $12/13^{th}$ of an equal volume of water.

[N.B. Density of proof spirit = 12/13 of density of water at 51^0F = 0.923 g/ml]

The US System: **Proof spirit** is 50% alcohol by volume (or 42.49% by weight).

The British / Indian system: **Proof spirit** is 57.1% ethanol by volume (or 48.24% by weight.

This means that any alcoholic solution that contains 57.1%v/v alcohol is a proof spirit and is said to be 100 proof.

100 degree proof alcohol = 57.1% v/v alcohol

If the strength of the alcohol is above 57.1%v/v alcohol, then the solution is called "*over proof*" (O.P).

If the strength of the alcohol is below 57.1%v/v alcohol, then the solution is called "*under proof*" (U.P).

Conversion factors: *Conversion of strength of alcohol from %v/v to **degrees proof** as per Indian system*

$$\text{Strength of alcohol} = \frac{\%v/v \text{ strength}}{57.1\%v/v} \times 100$$

*Conversion of strength of alcohol from **degrees proof** to %v/v as per Indian system*

$$\text{Strength of alcohol in \%v/v} = \frac{\text{Strength of alcohol in degree proof} \times 57.1}{100}$$

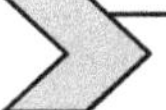 **Practice Examples**

Example 1: Find the strength of 95%v/v alcohol in terms of proof spirit.

$$\text{Strength of alcohol} = \frac{95\%v/v}{57.1\%v/v} \times 100 = 166.34 \text{ degree proof} = (166.34-100) \text{ degrees over proof} = 66.34^0 \text{ op}$$

Example 2: Find the strength of 20%v/v alcohol in terms of proof spirit.

$$\text{Strength of alcohol} = \frac{20\%v/v}{57.1\%v/v} \times 100 = 35.03 \text{ degree proof} = (100-35.03) \text{ degrees under proof} = 64.97^0 \text{ up}$$

Example 3: Calculate the real strength of 30^0op and 40^0up.

30^0op $= (100 + 30) = 130$ deg proof

Therefore the strength of alcohol $= \dfrac{130 \times 57.1}{100} = 74.23\%$v/v

40^0op $= (100 - 40) = 60$ deg proof

Therefore the strength of alcohol $= \dfrac{60 \times 57.1}{100} = 34.26\%$v/v

Example 4: How many proof gallons are contained in 5 gallon of 70%v/v alcohol?

1 proof gallon = 1 gallon proof alcohol = 1 gallon of 100 degrees proof alcohol

70% v/v alcohol $= \dfrac{70\%}{57.1\%} \times 100$ degrees proof alcohol

$= 122.59$ degrees proof alcohol

$= \dfrac{122.59}{100}$ proof alcohol $= 1.226$ proof alcohol

5 gallons 70%v/v alcohol = 5 gallons of 1.226 proof alcohol

$= 6.13$ proof gallon

Example 5: Convert 90%v/v alcohol into proof spirit

As 57.1 volume of ethyl alcohol = 100 volume of proof spirit

1 volume of ethyl alcohol = 100/57.1 = 1.7513 volume of proof spirit

90 volume of ethyl alcohol = 90 × 1.7513 volume of proof spirit

Hence Proof strength of 90% v/v alcohol = (90 × 1.7513) - 100 = 57.6°0/P

Similarly, Proof strength of 30% v/v alcohol can be calculated as follows.

Proof strength of 30%v/v alcohol = (30 × 1.7513) - 100 = -47.5 or 47.5°U/P

Thus 70 °0/P = 100 + 70/ 1.7513 =97% v/v of ethyl alcohol, and

70 °U/P = 100 - 70 / 1.7513 = 17.13% v/v of ethyl alcohol.

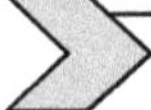

Iso-Osmotic and Isotonic Solutions

Iso-Osmotic: If a solution is placed in contact with membrane that is permeable to molecules of the solvent but not permeable to the molecules of the solute, the movement of the molecules of the solvent through the membrane is called *osmosis*. This type of membrane is called *semi-permeable* membrane. If a solution of a solute having higher concentration of the solute is placed on one side and solution of the same solute having low concentration of the same solute is placed on the other side of such a membrane, the solvent will tend to pass from the side containing lower solute concentration to the side containing higher solute concentration. This process will continue till an equilibrium with respect to solute concentration is established on both sides of the semi-permeable membrane.

Iso-osmotic: Body fluids like blood, lacrimal fluid, sebum etc. normally has an osmotic pressure that corresponds to the osmotic pressure exerted by 0.9% w/v solution of sodium chloride. Therefore, 0.9% w/v solution of sodium chloride is said to be iso-osmotic with physiologic fluids.

Isotonic: Isotonic means having the same tone. This term has reference to physiological compatibility. For example, a solution of boric acid that is iso-osmotic with both blood and lacrimal fluid is isotonic only with lacrimal fluid. This is because boric acid readily crosses the RBC membrane and causes hemolysis of these cells.

Iso-osmotic is a physical term that compares the osmotic pressure or other colligative properties of two liquids neither of which may be a physiologic fluid or which may behave as a physiologic fluid under a given set of conditions. A solution can be isotonic with a living cell only when there is no net gain or loss of water by the cell, or another change in the cell. Physiologic solutions with an osmotic pressure lower than that of body fluids, or 0.9% w/v sodium chloride solution are referred to as being *hypotonic*. Physiologic solutions having a greater pressure than the body fluids or 0.9% w/v sodium chloride solution are termed *hypertonic*.

Isotonicity: A solution is isotonic with a living cell if there is no net gain or loss of water by the cell, when it is in contact with this solution.

If a living cell is kept in contact with a solution and there is no loss or gain of water by the cell then the solution is said to be *isotonic* with the *cell*.

- It is found that the osmotic pressure of 0.9%w/v NaCl solution is same as blood plasma. So 0.9%w/v NaCl solution is *isotonic* with plasma.

  Tonicity– A. Isotonic – When a solution has same osmotic pressure as that of 0.9%w/v NaCl solution.

  B. Paratonic – Not isotonic

  (a) Hypotonic – The osmotic pressure of the solution is higher than 0.9% w/v NaCl solution

  (b) Hypertonic – The osmotic pressure of the solution is lower than 0.9% w/v NaCl solution

Test of tonicity

A red blood corpuscle is placed in a solution and after some time it is viewed under microscope.

Observation	Conclusion	Mechanism
The shape and size of the cell remained unchanged	The solution is isotonic	Osmotic pressure of the cell fluid and the solution are same. No movement of water occurs across the cell membrane.
The size of the cell increased and may burst.	The solution is hypotonic.	Osmotic pressure of the cell fluid is more than the solution. Water molecules moved from the solution to the interior of the cell, so the cell swelled.
The size of the cell is reduced or shrinked.	The solution is hypertonic.	Osmotic pressure of the cell fluid is less than the solution outside. Water molecule moved from the interior of the cell to the solution.

N.B. If the red blood cell bursts then the hemoglobin comes out of the cell and the plasma become red in color. This phenomenon is called haemolysis.

Importance of adjustment of tonicity in pharmaceutical dosage forms

1. *Solution for intravenous injection*: The injection must be isotonic with plasma, otherwise the red blood corpuscle may be haemolysed.

2. *Solution for subcutaneous injection*: Isotonicity is required but not essential, because the solution is coming in contact with fatty tissue and not in contact with blood.

3. *Solution for intramuscular injection*: The aqueous solution may be slightly hypertonic. This will draw water from the adjoining tissue and increase the absorption of the drug.

4. *Solution for intracutaneous injection*: Diagnostic preparations must be isotonic, because a paratonic solution may cause a false reaction.

5. *Solutions for intrathecal injection*: Intrathecal injections are introduced in the cavities of brain and spinal chord. It mixes with the cerebrospinal fluid (CSF). The volume of CSF is only 60 to 80ml. So a small volume of paratonic injection may change the osmotic pressure of the CSF, which may lead to vomiting and other side effects.

6. *Solutions for nasal drops*: Aqueous solutions applied within the nostril may produce irritation if it is paratonic. So nasal drops must be isotonic with plasma.

7. *Solutions for ophthalmic use*: Only one or two drops of ophthalmic solutions are generally used. So it is not essential for eyedrops to be isotonic. Slight paratonicity will not produce great irritation because the eyedrops will be diluted with the lachrymal fluid.

Calculations for adjustment of tonicity

N.B. It is difficult and time consuming to determine the osmotic pressure of a solution. So some indirect methods are adopted to compare between two isotonic solutions. Two solutions will produce same osmotic pressure if both contain the same numbers of *ultimate units*. These units may be as follows:

✓ These units may be molecules in case of substances those do not ionize.

✓ These units may be ions in case of substances those ionize.

✓ These units may be both ions and unionized molecules in case of weak electrolytes.

Some physical properties of these solutions depend on this number (or, collection) of units, such as osmotic pressure, freezing point depression (ΔT_f), vapor pressure etc. – these physical properties are called *colligative properties* of the solutions.

Since these colligative properties are inter-dependent, so osmotic pressures of two solutions can be compared from their colligative properties like freezing point depression.

Tonicity of a solution can be adjusted by the following methods:

1. Freezing point depression method (ΔT_f)
2. Sodium chloride equivalent method (E)
3. Isotonic solution V-Value method

OSMOL: It is the weight in grams of a solute existing in a solution as molecules (and / or ions, macromolecules, aggregates, etc), which is osmotically equivalent to a mole of an ideally behaving nonelectrolyte. Hence, the osmol weight of a nonelectrolyte in a dilute solution is equal to its gram molecular weight. Therefore, 1 osmol will be the amount of solute that will provide 1 Avogardo's number (6.023×10^{23}) particles in solution. It is also the amount of solute that on dissolution in 1 Kg water will produce an osmotic pressure increase of 17,000 torr at 0ºC or 19,300 torr at 37ºC.

Example: **For Nonelectrolyte - Dextrose**

1 mol of anhydrous dextrose = 180 g

1 osmol of anhydrous dextrose (nonelectrolyte) = 180 g

Therefore, 180 mg of anhydrous dextrose dissolved in 1 Kg water will produce an increase in osmotic pressure of 19.3 torr at 37ºC (body temperature).

For electrolyte – Sodium chloride

1 molecule of sodium chloride will produce one sodium and one chloride ion.

Therefore, 1 mol represents 2 osmol of sodium chloride.

Hence, 1 osmol Sodium chloride = 58.5 g / 2 = 29.25 g

Therefore, 29.25 = 6.023×10^{23} ions (particles)

Osmolality & Osmolarity

Osmolality:

1 osmolal concentration = 1 osmol of solute / Kg of water

Osmolal solutions represent a w/w relationship between the solute and solvent.

Example: **For nonelectrolyte - Dextrose**

An osmol of any nonelectrolyte is equivalent to 1 mol of that compound, therefore, 1 osmolal solution of a nonelectrolyte is equal to its 1 molal solution.

For ionizing electrolyte – Sodium chloride

1 osmol = 0.5 mol of sodium chloride

Therefore, 1 osmolal solution of sodium chloride = 0.5 molal solution

Osmolarity:

1 osmolar solution = 1 osmol of solute per 1 L of solution.

Osmolar solutions represent a w/v relationship between solute and solvent.

Example: **For nonelectrolyte - Dextrose**

1 osmolar = 1 molar solution

For ionizing electrolyte – Sodium chloride

1 osmolar solution will contain 1 osmol of sodium chloride per liter which will be a 0.5 molar solution.

NOTE: A 1 osmolar solution of a solute will always be more concentrated than a 1 osmolal solution.

Calculation of Osmolarity

$$\text{Osmolarity} \left(\frac{mOsmol}{L} \right) = \frac{g}{L} \times \frac{mols}{g} \times \frac{osmol}{mol} \times \frac{1000\,mOsmol}{osmol}$$

The number of osmol / mol is equal to 1 for nonelectrolytes and is equal to number of ions per molecule for strong electrolytes.

0.9% sodium chloride has an osmolar concentration of 308 mOsmol/L and a concentration of 154 mOsmol/L in either sodium or chloride ion.

2. $$\frac{gwater}{mLsolution} = \frac{gsolution}{mLsolution} - \frac{gsolute}{mLsolution}$$

Then, Osmolarity

$$\left(\frac{mOsmol}{Lsolution}\right) = osmolality\left(\frac{mOsmol}{1000gwater}\right) \times \left(\frac{gwater}{mLsolution}\right)$$

Osmolality depends on the number of particles in the solution. The number of particles, in turn, influence the colligative properties of a solution namely osmotic pressure elevation, boiling point elevation, vapor pressure depression and freezing point depression.

Methods of Adjusting Tonicity

1. Freezing point depression method

The freezing point of normal, healthy human blood is $-0.52°C$. This means that in water as medium, any suspended or dissolved solute that freezes at $-0.52°C$ will be isotonic with blood. Also, it is known that 0.9% w/v solution produces freezing point depression of 0.52 °C. Therefore, a 0.9% w/v solution of sodium chloride is isotonic with human blood, serum, lacrimal fluid etc.

The Tables available in the literature list "D" values of many solutes. The "D" value has units of °C/y% drug. For example, a   "D" value of 0.05°/ 0.5% drug means that the drug will produce a freezing point depression of 0.05°C when used at a concentration of 0.5% w/v. "D" value is nearly proportional to concentration.

Example 1   Dexamethasone sodium phosphate   0.1%

Purified water qs   30 mL

"D" value given is $0.050° / 0.5\%$

A. Contribution of 0.1% drug towards freezing point depression will be:

(0.050 x 0.1) / 0.5 = 0.010°C

Freezing point depression of human blood = 0.52°C

Freezing point depression remaining to be contributed by adding sodium chloride = 0.52 – 0.010 = 0.51 °C

0.9% w/v sodium chloride provides freezing point depression of 0.52°C

Therefore, 0.51°C depression in freezing point will be provided by (0.9 x 0.51) / 0.52 = 0.883% sodium chloride

For 30 mL solution the amount of sodium chloride needed will be (0.883 x 30) / 100 = 0.265 g sodium chloride

(B) If this solution has to be made isotonic by adding dextrose ("D" value = 0.091°C/1%)

Then, 0.091 °C freezing point depression will be provided by 1% dextrose

Therefore, 0.51°C depression will be provided by: (0.51 x 1) / 0.091 = 5.6% dextrose

For 100 mL the quantity of dextrose required is 5.6g

Therefore, for 30 mL solution, the quantity of dextrose required will be: (5.6 x 30) / 100 = 1.68g dextrose

Hence, 1.68g dextrose can be added instead of 0.265g sodium chloride to make this solution isotonic.

2. Sodium chloride equivalent method

This method uses "E" value listed in the literature. "E" value is the weight of sodium chloride that will produce the same osmotic effect as 1g of the drug. For example, a "E" value of 0.18 means 0.18g of sodium chloride can produce the same osmotic effect as 1g of drug.

Example 1	Dexamethasone sodium phosphate	0.1%
	Purified water qs	30 mL

"E" value given is 0.18

A. Total quantity of drug in formulation will be: (30 x 0.1) / 100 = 0.03g

Total quantity of sodium chloride required for 30 mL if there was no drug = (30 x 0.9) / 100 = 0.27g

Contribution of drug in terms of sodium chloride: (0.18 x 0.03) / 1 = 0.0054g

Therefore, quantity of sodium chloride required to make 30 mL solution isotonic = 0.27 – 0.0054 = 0.265g

B. If this solution has to be made isotonic by adding dextrose ("E" value = 0.16)

0.16g sodium chloride is equivalent to 1g drug in terms of isotonicity

0.265g sodium chloride will be equivalent to: (0.265 x 1) / 0.16 = 1.66 dextrose

Hence, 1.66g dextrose can be added instead of 0.265g sodium chloride to make this solution isotonic.

3. Molecular concentration method

At normal temperature and pressure a solution containing 1 g molecule of a non-ionizing solute in 22.4 L has an osmotic pressure of 1 atmosphere.

This means that a solution containing 1 g molecule in 1 L (molar solution) will have an osmotic pressure of 22.4 atmosphere.

Osmotic pressure of blood plasma is 6.7 atmosphere

Therefore, molarity of plasma = 6.7 / 22.4 = 0.3M

Hence, 0.3M solution of any non-ionizing solute will be iso-osmotic with plasma.

For ionizing solutes, iso-osmoticity can be calculated by 0.3M / N, where 'N' is the number of ions.

pH AND BUFFER SOLUTIONS

A proton binds with a molecule of water to produce a hydronium ion, i.e. $H_2O + H^+ = H_3O^+$.

Mathematically the pH of a solution is defined as the negative logarithm of hydrogen ion (more appropriately hydronium $H_3O^{+)}$ concentration in **molarity**.

$$pH = - \log [H_3O^+]$$

Buffer / buffer solution / buffered solution refer to the ability of an aqueous solution to resist a change of pH on adding acid or alkali, or on dilution with a solvent.

N.B. Distilled water has very little buffer action, hence carbon dioxide of air, when equilibrated with distilled water (pH = 7.0), the pH of the water changes to 5.7.

A solution will show buffer action if a conjugate acid-base pair is present in the solution.

e.g.

$$CH_3COOH + H_2O \rightleftharpoons CH_3COO^- + H_3O^+$$

| Weak acid | Weak base | Strong base | Strong acid |

The dissociation constant, $Ka = \dfrac{[CH_3COO^-][H_3O^+]}{[CH_3COOH]}$

Taking logarithm of both hand sides we get,

$$\log Ka = \log [CH_3COO^-] + \log [H_3O^+] - \log [CH_3COOH]$$

Multiplying -1 with both hand sides yield:

$$- \log Ka = - \log [H_3O^+] + \log [CH_3COOH] - \log [CH_3COO^-]$$

or, $pKa = pH + \log [CH_3COOH] - \log [CH_3COO^-]$

or, $pH = pKa - \log [CH_3COOH] + \log [CH_3COO^-]$

or, $pH = pKa + \log \dfrac{[CH_3COO^-]}{[CH_3COOH]}$

or, $pH = pKa + \log \dfrac{[base]}{[acid]}$

This equation is called **Henderson-Hasselbalch equation.**

This ratio of $\dfrac{[base]}{[acid]}$ and Ka determines the pH of the solution. For a certain weak acid or base Ka is constant, so if the ratio of concentrations of the [base] / [acid] is changed the pH of the buffer solution can be changed.

This equation can be used in the following buffer systems:

Name of the buffer system	Conjugate acid	Conjugate base
Acetic acid – Sodium acetate buffer	Acetic acid (CH_3COOH)	Acetate ion (CH_3COO^-)
Ammonia – Ammonium chloride buffer	Ammonium ion (NH_4^+)	Ammonia (NH_3)
Monosodium phosphate – Disodium phosphate	Monosodium phosphate (NaH_2PO_4)	Disodium phosphate (Na_2HPO_4)
Phenobarbital – Sodium phenobarbital	Phenobarbital	Sodium phenobarbital

Use of Henderson – Hasselbalch equation

1. The pH of a buffer solution can be calculated if the pKa, concentration of the base and acid are known.

2. During preparation of a buffer solution the ratio of the concentration of the conjugate acid and base pair can be calculated.

3. To calculate the buffer capacity of a buffer solution.

Example 1: *What will be the pH of a solution containing acetic acid and sodium acetate, each in 0.1M concentration? Ka of acetic acid is 1.8 x 10⁻⁵ at 25⁰C.*

Ans: $pKa = -\log Ka = -\log 1.8 \times 10^{-5}. = -(\log 1.8 + \log 10^{-5}) = -(0.26 - 5)$
$= -(-4.74) = 4.74$

Concentration of acid = [acid] = $[CH_3COOH]$ = 0.1M

Concentration of base = [base] = $[CH_3COO^-]$ = 0.1 M

From Hender- Hasselbalch equation we get

$$pH = pKa + \log \frac{[base]}{[acid]} = 4.74 + \log \frac{0.1}{0.1} = 4.74 + \log 1 = 4.74 + 0 = 4.74 \; Ans.$$

Example 2: *An acetic acid- acetate buffer is to be prepared having pH 4.5. What will be the ratio of the molar concentration of the acid base pair. Given pKa of acetic acid = 4.74.*

Ans: Using Henderson – Hasselbalch equation we get:

$$pH = pKa + \log\frac{[base]}{[acid]} \qquad or, \quad pH - pKa = \log\frac{[base]}{[acid]}$$

or, $\quad \dfrac{[base]}{[acid]} =$ antilog (pH $-$ pKa) $= 10^{(pH - pKa)} = 10^{(4.5 - 4.74)} = 10^{-0.24} = 0.575$

The answer is [sodium acetate]:[acetic acid] = 0.575: 1

Buffer Capacity

The ability of a buffer solution to resist changes in pH upon addition of acid or alkali is measured in terms of *buffer capacity* of the solution.

Van Slyke has defined the *buffer capacity* as follows:

The amount (gm-equivalent) of strong acid or strong base, required to be added to a solution to change its pH by 1 unit.

In mathematical form: *Buffer capacity of a solution =*

$$\frac{gm\ eq\ of\ a\ strong\ acid\ or\ strong\ alkali\ added}{change\ of\ pH}$$

Example 3: *(a) What is the change of pH on adding 0.01mol of NaOH to 1 L of 0.10 M acetic acid? (b)Calculate the buffer capacity of the acetic solution. Ka = 1.75 x 10⁻⁴.*

Ans:

(a)   Calculation of pH of 0.1 M solution of acetic acid

$$[H_3O^+] = \sqrt{Ka[CH_3COOH]} = \sqrt{1.75 \times 10^{-4} \times 0.1} = 4.18 \times 10^{-3}.$$

Therefore pH $= - \log (4.18 \times 10^{-3}) = - (-2.38) = 2.38$

(b)   On adding 0.01moles of NaOH, 0.01 mol of acetic acid will be converted to form 0.01 mol of acetic acid.

So after addition of NaOH $[CH_3COO^-] = 0.01$mol/ L $= 0.01$M

$\qquad [CH_3COOH] = (0.10$mol $- 0.01$mol$)/L = 0.09$ mol / L $= 0.09$ M

Applying Henderson – Hasselbalch equation to calculate the pH of the final solution we get:

$$\text{pH} = \text{pKa} + \log\frac{[\text{base}]}{[\text{acid}]} = 4.76 + \log\frac{[0.01]}{[0.09]} = 4.76 + (-0.954) = 3.81$$

Therefore the change in pH after addition of NaOH = final pH $-$ initial pH = $3.81 - 2.38 = 1.43$

So, from definition the

Buffer capacity of the solution =

$$\frac{\text{eqwt of NaOH added}}{\text{change in pH}} = \frac{\text{mols of NaOH added}}{\text{change in pH}} = \frac{0.01}{1.43} = 0.007 \ Ans.$$

Example 4: *(a) What is the change of pH on adding 0.01mol of NaOH to 1 L of buffer solution of 0.10 M acetic acid 0.1M of sodium acetate? (b)Calculate the buffer capacity of the solution. Ka = 1.75 x 10⁻⁴.*

Ans:

(a)   The pH of the buffer solution before addition of NaOH is

[base] $=$ [CH$_3$COO$^-$] $= 0.1$M

[acid] $=$ [CH$_3$COOH] $= 0.1$ M

$$\text{pH} = \text{pKa} + \log\frac{[\text{base}]}{[\text{acid}]} = 4.76 + \log\frac{[0.1]}{[0.1]} = 4.76 + \log(1) = 4.76 + 0 = 4.76$$

(b)   On adding 0.01mol of NaOH per litre to this buffer solution 0.01mol aicd will be converted to base:

[base] $=$ [CH$_3$COO$^-$] $= (0.10\text{mol} + 0.01\text{mol}) / \text{L} = 0.11\text{mol} / \text{L} = 0.11$ M

[acid] $=$ [CH$_3$COOH] $= (0.10\text{mol} - 0.01\text{mol}) / \text{L} = 0.09 \text{ mol/L} = 0.09$ M

$$\text{pH} = \text{pKa} + \log\frac{[\text{base}]}{[\text{acid}]} = 4.76 + \log\frac{[0.11]}{[0.09]} = 4.76 + \log(1.22) = 4.76 +$$

$0.09 = 4.85$

Therefore the change in pH after addition of NaOH = final pH $-$ initial pH = $4.85 - 4.76 = 0.09$

So, from definition the

Buffer capacity of the solution =

$$\frac{\text{eqwt of NaOH added}}{\text{change in pH}} = \frac{\text{mols of NaOH added}}{\text{change in pH}} = \frac{0.01}{0.09} = 0.111 \ Ans.$$

So, this buffer solution has greater buffer capacity (0.111) than the solution in problem-3 (0.007).

Calculations Based on Radioisotopes

Disintegration Rate of a Radioisotope

Radioisotope nucleus $\rightarrow$ Daughter nucleus

The rate at which the radio-isotopes are degrading $= \dfrac{dN}{dt}$	where, N is the number of radioactive nuclei left to be disintegrated at time t
It is found that the degradation follows first order kinetics, i.e. $\dfrac{dN}{dt} = \lambda N$,	where λ = decay constant of the radionucleide

So, $\dfrac{dN}{dt} = \lambda N$ or, $\dfrac{dN}{N} = \lambda\, dt$

Integrating both sides we get

$$\int_{N_0}^{N} \frac{dN}{N} = \lambda \int_{0}^{t} dt \quad \text{or,} \quad [\ln N]_{N_0}^{N} = \lambda(t-0) \text{ or, } \ln N = \ln N_0 - \lambda t \text{ or, } \ln\frac{N}{N_0} = -\lambda t$$

or, $N/N_0 = e^{-\lambda t}$ or, $N = N_0 e^{-\lambda t}$

N_0 = initial number of radioactive nuclei

N = number of radioactive nuclei at time t

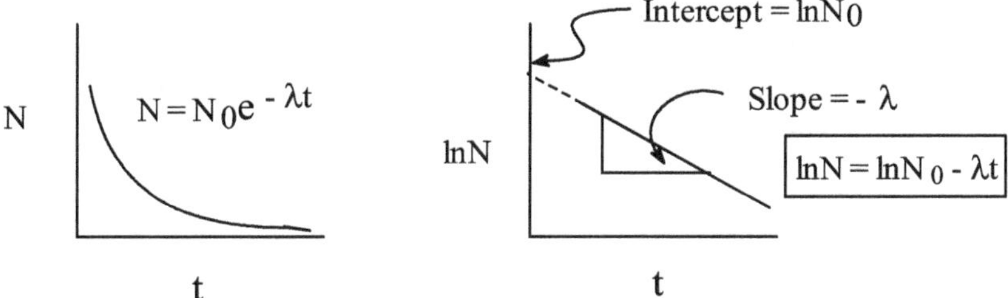

Half-life of radioactive nuclei

The time taken for half of the radioactive nuclei to disintegrate (i.e. for the activity to fall to half of its original value) is known as the half-life ($t_{1/2}$)

At time, $t = 0$ $N = N_0$.

At time, $t = t_{1/2}$ $N = N_0/2$

Therefore, $\ln\dfrac{N}{N_0} = -\lambda t$,   or, $\ln\dfrac{N_0/2}{N_0} = -\lambda t_{1/2}$

or, $\ln(1/2) = -\lambda\, t_{1/2}$.or, $-\ln 2 = -\lambda\, t_{1/2}$.   or, $t_{1/2} = \dfrac{0.693}{\lambda}$

Units of radioactivity

One g of radium was selected as the unit of radioactivity and was called *Curie*.

From 1 *curie* (Ci) radium 3.7×10^{10} numbers of nuclei disintegrates per second.

So   1 Ci = 3.7×10^{10} *dnps*   *dnps* = disintegrating nucleus per second

Example:

The activity of a sample solution of ^{131}I was 500 µCi (microcurie) /ml at noon on Monday. Calculate its activity at 4.0 p.m. on Thursday. (Half-life of ^{131}I = 8days)

Solution: $t_{1/2}$ = 8 days = 8 x 24 hours = 192 hours

From equation, $t_{1/2} = \dfrac{0.693}{\lambda}$, we get $\lambda = \dfrac{0.693}{t_{1/2}} = \dfrac{0.693}{192\,hr} = 0.00361\ hr^{-1}$.

From equation $lnN = lnN_0 - \lambda t$

In this problem $N_0 = 500$ µCi /ml

t = the time from 12 noon Monday to 4 p.m. Thursday = $3 \times 24 + 4 = 76$ hrs

$\therefore lnN \quad = ln\,500 - 0.00361 \times 76$

$= 6.218 - 0.2743$

$= 5.994$

or, $N = e^{5.994} = 381..1$

Ans. At 4 p.m. Thursday the radioactivity will be 381.1 µCi / ml.

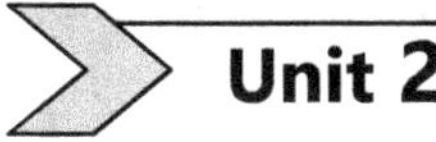

Unit 2

Liquid Dosage Forms

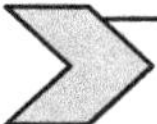

Solubility and its Expression

When a solid solute is dissolved in a liquid solvent two types of interactions occur

(i) the intra-molecular force between the solute molecules;

(ii) the intermolecular force between the solute and solvent molecules.

When a solute dissolve, the substance's intra-molecular forces (cohesive force) must be overcome by the force of attraction between the solute and solvent molecules (adhesive force).

Expression of Solubility (I.P)

Terminology	Approximate quantities (ml) of solvent by volume for 1 part (1 gm) of solute by weight
Very soluble	less than 1 part
Freely soluble	from 1 to 10 parts
Soluble	from 10 to 30 parts
Sparingly soluble	from 30 to 100 parts
Slightly soluble	from 100 to 1000 parts
Very slightly soluble	from 1000 to 10,000 parts
Practically insoluble	more than 10,000 parts

Solubility

The *solubility* of an agent in a particular solvent indicates the *maximum* concentration to which a solution may be prepared with that agent and that solvent.

Determination of Equilibrium Solubility of a Drug

An excess of the drug (finely powdered to minimize the time required to attain the equilibrium) is placed in a vial along with a specific amount of the solvent. The tightly closed vial is then agitated at constant temperatures (preferably at temperature somewhat higher than room temperature e.g. 30^0C so that constant conditions can be maintained regardless of normal laboratory temperature variations), and the amount of drug in solution is determined periodically by assay of a filtered sample of the supernate. Equilibrium is not achieved until at least two successive samplings give the same result.

The *solubility* is generally expressed in mg of solute per ml of solvent at 25^0 C or per 100 ml etc.

Solubility of a drug depends on temperature, solvent, pH and the chemical nature of the molecule itself. By modifying these parameters, the solubility of a drug can be manipulated according to the requirement of designing the dosage form.

pH

A large number of drugs are either weak acids or weak bases. The solubility of these agents can be markedly influenced by the pH of the environment. When a weakly acidic drug is dissolved in water it can remain in three states, namely undissolved, dissolved and ionized which can be expressed in the following reaction format:

$$\text{DH (solid)} \rightleftharpoons \text{DH (solution)} \rightleftharpoons \text{D}^- + \text{H}^+$$

DH (solid) — (Undissolved)
DH (solution) — (Undissociated)
D⁻ (Dissociated / ionized) + H⁺ (Proton)

The relationship between equilibrium solubility of a weakly acidic drug and the pH of the environment can be expressed by Henderson-Hasselbach equation:

$$pH = pKa + \log \frac{[D^-]}{[DH]}$$

where

pKa = Dissociation constant of the acid

$[D^-]$ = Molar concentration of ionized drug

[DH] = Molar concentration of unionized drug

The same equation can be written in the following forms:

$$pH = pKa + \log \frac{[\text{ionized}]}{[\text{unionized}]}$$

$$pH = pKa + \log \frac{[\text{base}]}{[\text{acid}]}$$

where   DH = Acid

   D^- = Corresponding base of the acid (DH)

Weak Acid	Weak Base
DH (solid) ⇌ DH(solution) ⇌ D⁻ + H⁺ Dissolved Unionised $pH = pKa + \log \dfrac{[D^-]}{[DH]}$ $pH = pKa + \log \dfrac{[ionised]}{[unionised]}$ $pH = pKa + \log \dfrac{[base]}{[acid]}$ DH = acid D⁻ = corresponding base of DH	DOH (solid) ⇌ DOH(solution) ⇌ D⁺ + OH⁻ Dissolved Unionised $pH = pKa + \log \dfrac{[DOH^-]}{[D^+]}$ $pH = pKa + \log \dfrac{[unionised]}{[ionised]}$ $pH = pKa + \log \dfrac{[base]}{[acid]}$ DOH = base D⁺ = corresponding acid of the base DOH

To maintain the drug in soluble state, the solution of a drug must be done in a suitable buffer solution. The buffer must have the following properties:

1. The buffer must have adequate capacity in the desired pH range.
2. The buffer must be biologically safe for the intended use.
3. The buffer (or its pH range) must have minimum interference on the stability of the final product.
4. The buffer should permit acceptable flavoring and coloring of the product.

e.g. Some commonly used buffer systems are ammonium chloride, diethanol amine, triethanolamine, boric acid, carbonic acid, phosphate buffer, glutamic acid, tartaric acid, citric acid buffer, acetic acid buffer etc.

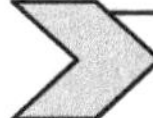 ## Cosolvency

Weak electrolytes and nonpolar molecules frequently have poor water solubility. These types of solutes are more soluble in a mixture of solvents than in one solvent alone. This phenomenon is known as cosolvency; and the solvents that, in combination increase the solubility of the solute are called cosolvents.

To increase the water solubility of a drug, another water miscible solvent in which the drug has good solubility is mixed.

Mechanism of action

It has been proposed that a cosolvent system works by reducing the interfacial tension between the predominantly aqueous solutions and the hydrophobic solute.

Examples of commonly used cosolvents

Ethanol, sorbitol, glycerin, propylene glycol and several members of the polyethylene glycol polymer (PEG200) series are the limited number of cosolvents of water those are used and are acceptable in oral preparation.

Use of cosolvents

Cosolvents are used to increase the solubility of weak electrolytes, non-polar molecules and volatile constituents used to impart a desirable flavor and odour to the product.

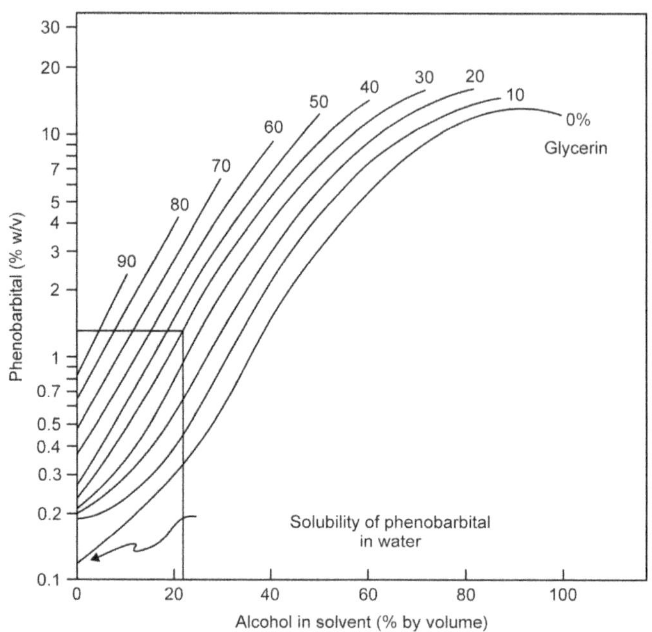

The solubility of Phenobarbital in a mixture of water, alcohol, and glycerin.

Approximately 1 g of phenobarbital is soluble in 1000 ml of water, in 10 ml of alcohol, in 40 ml of chloroform, and in 15 ml of ether. Solubility enhances with increase in the concentration of glycerin. For example, at 22% alcohol, 40% glycerin, and the remainder water (38%), 1.5% w/v of Phenobarbital is dissolved. The solubility of phenobarbital in water-alcohol-glycerin mixtures depicted the above mentioned.

Dielectric Constant

One property of a solvent system is its dielectric constant. The dielectric constant of a solvent can be defined as the ratio of the capacitances of a capacitor filled with the solvent and air respectively.

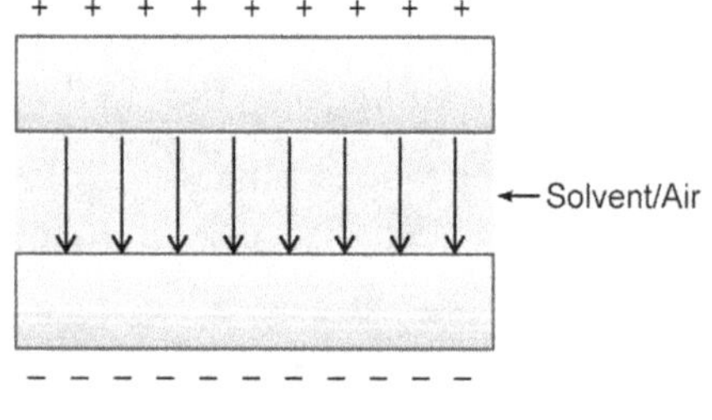

$$\text{Diectric constant } (\varepsilon) = \frac{C_{Solvent}}{C_{air}}$$

where, C is the capacitance of the condenser filled with respective medium (solvent or air) e.g dielectric constant of water is 78.5

Every solute shows a maximum solubility in any given solvent system, at one or more specific dielectric constants.

The purpose is to determine the relationship between solubility of a solute with dielectric constant(s) at which maximum solubility is attained.

Pharmaceutical formulations of comparable dielectric constant can thus be prepared, and the most appropriate solvent system can be selected on the basis of solubility, stability and organoleptic requirements.

Solubilization

The spontaneous increase of solubility of poorly water-soluble solute molecules into an aqueous solution of surface-active agents (or surfactants) in which a thermodynamically stable solution is formed, is called solubilization.

Mechanism

When surfactants are added to water at low concentrations, they tend to orient at the air-liquid interface.

As additional surfactant is added, the interface becomes fully occupied, and the excess molecules get oriented into the bulk of the liquid.

At still higher concentrations, the molecules of surfactant in the bulk of the liquid begin to form oriented aggregates or micelles. This change in orientation occurs suddenly.

The concentration of surface active agent at which micelle formation occurs is called critical micelle concentration.

Solubilization is thought to occur due to the solute dissolving in or being adsorbed onto the micelle. The water solubility of the solute increases with increase in the concentration of the micelles.

Examples of some solubilizing agents:

Polyoxyethylene 20 sorbitan monooleate

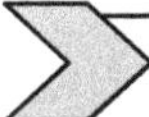

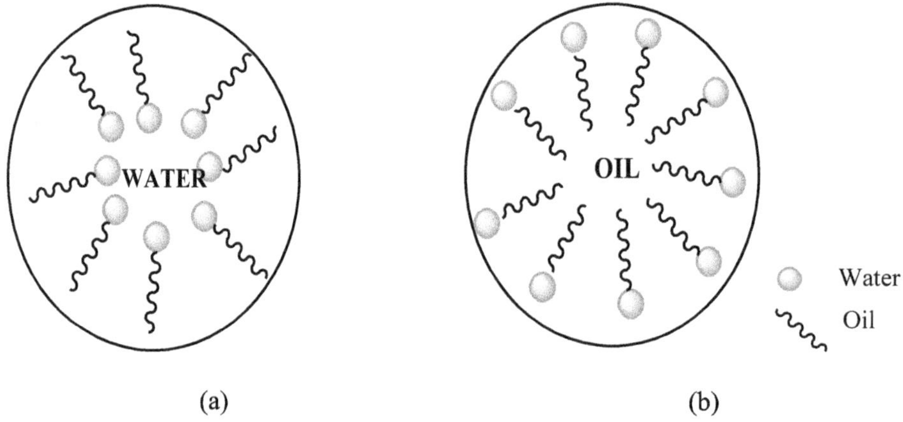

It has generally been found that surface-active-agents having HLB (Hydrophilic Lipophilic Balance) values higher than 15 acts better as solubilizing agents.

(a)   (b)

Fig. 2.2 (a) w/o type of emulsion, (b) o/w type of emulsion

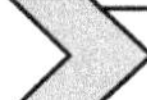 **Complexation**

Solubility of a compound may be increased by complexing with a complexing agent. e.g. solubility of para amino benzoic acid (PABA) may be increased by complexing with caffeine.

When an insoluble compound forms a complex which is more soluble in the solvent - the total solubility is equal to the inherent solubility of the uncomplexed drug plus the concentration of drug-complex in solution.

When a certain amount of drug is mixed in water some amount will get dissolved (A) and some amount will remain undissolved. If a complexing agent is added to it some drug will be complexed and become soluble in water. Hence, the total solubility of the drug increases.

When more complexing agent is added total solubility will increase; at a certain concentration of complexing agent the solution will become saturated with respect to free drug and the complex (B). After this point, if more complexing agent is used, the remaining drug (undissolved) will form complex and the excess complex will be precipitated (C). When no drug is left for complexation, complexes of higher order may be formed.

e.g. I_2 is sparingly soluble in water. To dissolve it KI (potassium iodide) is added which makes a complex $KI.I_2$ (i.e. KI_3). After (C) it forms KI. $2I_2$, $KI.3I_2$ etc.

Hydrotrophy

The term hydrotrophy has been used to designate the increase in solubility in water of various substances due to the presence of large amounts of additives.

Mechanism of action

Some workers have speculated that this phenomenon is more closely related to complexation involving a weak interaction between the hydrotrophic agent and the solute.

Another view is that the phenomenon could be due to change in solvent character because of the large amount of additive is needed to bring about the increase in solubility.

Examples

Since a large concentration of hydrotrophic agent is required (in the range of 20 to 50%) to produce a modest increase in solubility, its pharmaceutical applications are very less.

S.No.	Drug	Hydrotrophic agent	Structures
1.	Benzoic acid	Sodium benzoate	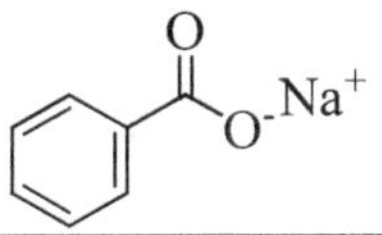
2.	Theophylline	Sodium acetate and sodium glycinate	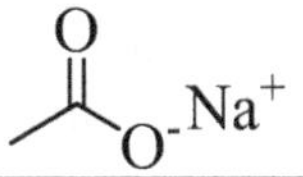
3.	Iodine	Polyvinyl pyrrolidone (PVP)	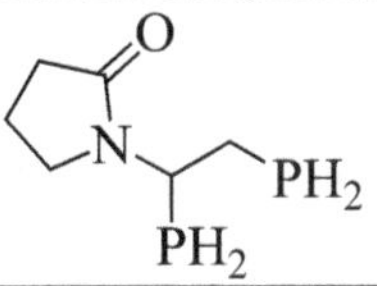
4.	Adrenochrome mono semicarbazone	Sodium salicylate	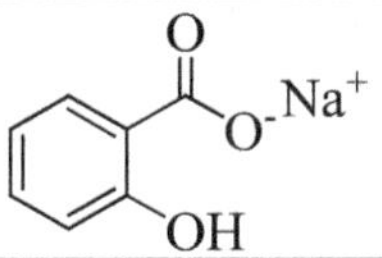

Additives and Solvents for Oral Preparations

Several non-pharmacological pharmaceutical additives, excipients and solvents (organic and inorganic) are widely employed in the solid dosage forms as well as oral liquid preparations. These include vehicles (e.g. purified water, ethanol, glycerin, propylene glycol), sweetners (e.g. glycerol, sucrose), colourants (e.g. Amaranth, tartrazine), flavoring agents (e.g. lemon spirit, raspberry syrup) and preservatives (e.g. benzoic acid, cinnamic acid). Some of the significant additives commonly used in pharmaceutical dispensing laboratory are summarized as below:

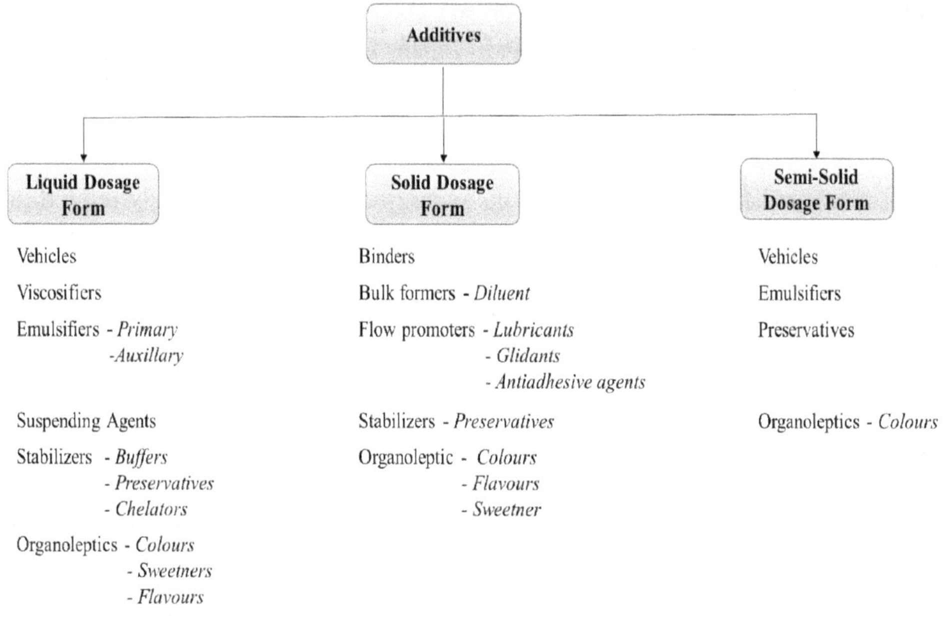

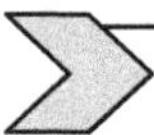 ## Types of Pharmaceutical Grade Water
Purified Water (USP)

Naturally occurring water exerts its solvent effect on most substances. In oral preparations the water used is potable water or Purified Water USP.

Specifications of Purified Water USP	
Method of preparations:	By distillation or by ion-exchange.
Total solid:	Less than 10 parts per million (ppm)
pH:	Between 5 and 7.

Type	As per USP Standard	As per IP Standard
Purified water	Purified water is water obtained by suitable process. It is obtained from water complying with the u.s. Environment protection agency national primary drinking water regulation or with the drinking water regulation of eu, japan or with the who's drinking water quality guidelines. It contains no added substance. (complies with usp test for conductivity and total organic carbon).	Purified water is water suitable for pharmaceutical use by processes such as distillation, ionexchange treatment (deionisation or demineralisation), or reverse osmosis. The minimal quality of source or feed water for the production of purified water is drinking water. The prepared water meets the specifications for chemical purity and it contains no added substances. (should be evaluated for sterility, microorganisms and other particulate matter depending upon the method of preparing it).
Water for injection	Water for injection is water purified by distillation or a purification process that is equivalent or superior to distillation in the removal of chemicals and microorganisms. It is obtained from water complying with the u.s. environment protection agency national primary drinking water regulation or with the drinking water regulation of eu, japan or with the who's drinking water quality guidelines. It contains no added substance. It is intended for use in preparation of parenteral solutions. Where used for the preparation of parenteral solutions subject to final sterilization, use suitable means to minimize microbial growth or first render the water for injection sterile and thereafter, protect it from microbial contamination. (it contains less than 0.25 usp endotoxin units per ml. Complies with usp test for total organic carbon and water conductivity).	Water for injections is water that is pre-treated to render it suitable for subsequent treatment and then purified by distillation or by reverse osmosis and it meets all of the chemical requirements stated under purified water. It is not intended to be sterile but should comply with the test for a limit of bacterial endotoxins, or as appropriate, with the test for pyrogens. It must be produced, stored and distributed under conditions designed to prevent production of endotoxins or pyrogens.

Contd....

Sterile water for injection	It is prepared from water for injection that is sterilized and suitably packaged. It contains no antimicrobial agent or other added substance. It should be preserved in single dose glass (type i or ii) or plastic containers of less than 1 l capacity. Label should indicate 'not for intravscular injection' because it has not been made isotonic. Ph should be between 5.0 – 7.0 in a solution containing 0.3 ml of saturated potassium chloride solution per 100 ml of test solution. It contains less than 0.25 usp endotoxin units per ml. It should meet the requirements for usp sterility and particulate matter. Should meet the requirements for ammonia, calcium, chloride, carbon dioxide and sulfate.	It is sterilised within 12 hours of collection and distributed in sterile containers. It is intended mainly for use as a solvent for parenteral preparations such as powders for injection that are distributed dry because of limited stability of their solutions. It should be packaged only in single dose containers of not larger than 1-litre size
Sterile water for irrigation	It is prepared from sterile water for injection that is sterilized and suitably packaged. It contains no antimicrobial agent or other added substance. It should be preserved in single dose glass 9type i or ii) or plastic containers and may contain a volume of more than 1l and may be designed to empty rapidly. Label 'for irrigation only' and 'not for injection'. It should comply with the usp tests as described for sterile water for injection.	Not available
Bacteriostatic water for injection	This is water for injection to which one or more suitable antimicrobial preservatives have been added. It is intended to be used as a diluent in parenteral products that require repeated content withdrawls	This is usually water for injections which may have been sterilised. It is free from a level of endotoxin that would yield any detectable reaction or interference with the lysate used in the test for bacterial endotoxins.
Sterile purified water	It is the purified water that is packaged and rendered sterile. It is used in the preparaton of nonparentereal compedial dosage forms or in analytical applications requiring purified water where access to validated purified water system is not practical / where only a relatively small quantity is needed/ where sterile purified water is required/ where bulk packaged purified water is not suitably microbiologically controlled.	Not available

Contd....

Water for hemodialysis	It is prepared from purified water by further treatment to reduce the chemical and microbial components. (it should comply with the usp limits set for water for hemodialysis with microbial limits of 100 cfu per ml and endotoxin limit of 2 usp endotoxin units per ml using soybean-casein digest agar medium or equivalent at temperature ranging from 30-35 °c for nlt 48 hours.	Not available
Sterile water for inhalation	It is water for injection that is packaged and rendered sterile and is intended for use in inhalators and in preparationo of inhalation solution. It carries a less stringent specification for bacterial endotoxins than sterile water for injection and therefore is not suitable for pareteral applications	Not available
Pure steam	It is prepared from suitable pretreated source water, analogous to the pretreatment used for purified water or water for injection, vaporized with suitable mist elimination and distributed under pressure. It is intended for use in steam sterilization of equipment and in other processess such as cleaning where condensate would directly contact official articles, containers for these articles, process surfaces that would in turn contact these articles, or materials which are used in analyzing such articles, pure steam may be used for air humidificaiton in controlled manufacturing areas where offical articles or article contact surfaces are exposed to the resulting conditioned air.	It is intended for use in steam-sterilising porous loads and equipment and in other processes such as cleaning where condensate would directly contact the pharmacopoeial articles and containers for these articles process surfaces that would in turn contact these articles or materials that are used in testing such articles. Pure steam is prepared from suitably pretreated source water, similar to the pre-treatment used for purified water or water for injections, vaporised with a suitable mist elimination, and distribution under pressure. Sources of contamination during the preparation are entrained water droplets, anti-corrosion steam additives, or particulate matter from the production and distribution system.
Distilled water	It is produced by vaporizing liquid water and condensing it in a purer state. It is used primarily as a solvent for reagent preparation, but it is also specified in the execution of other aspects of tests, such as for rinsing an analyte, transferring a test material as a slurry, as a calibration standardor analytical blank, and for test apparatus cleaning. Also called as **starting water** to be used for making *high purity water.*	It is produced by vaporising water and condensing it in a purer state. It is mainly used for preparing reagents but may also be required for other laboratory operations such as rinsing an analyte, transferring a test material as slurry, as a calibration standard or analytical blank and for cleaning of apparatus. Unless specifically indicated, water meeting the requirements for purified water derived by other means of purification could be equally suitable where the use of distilled water is recommended.

Contd....

Freshly distilled water	Also called as **recently distilled water**. Produced in similar way as distilled water and should be used shortly after its generation. It ensures avoidance of endotoxin contamination as well as any other adventitious form of contamination from the air or containers that could arise with prolonged storage. Used for preparing subcutaneous test animal injections as well as for a reagent solvent tests for which there appears to be no particular high-water purity need that could be ascribed to being freshly distilled. (should comply with chemical, endotoxin and microbiological purity as for water for injection)	Also known as "recently distilled water", it is the article produced in a similar manner as distilled water but is to be used shortly after its generation. This implies the need to avoid endotoxin contamination, or any other adventitious forms of contamination from the air or containers that could arise with prolonged storage. It is used for preparing solutions for subcutaneous test animal injections and also for preparing specific reagent solutions.
Deionized water	It produced by ion exchange process in which the contamination ions are replaced with either H+ or OH– ions. Used as a solvent for reagent preparation, as calibration standard or analytical blank, and for test apparatus cleaning	It is produced by an ion-exchange process in which contaminating ions are replaced with either H+ or OH– ions. It is used primarily as a solvent for preparing reagents and for the other aforementioned laboratory operations where distilled water is used. In this case too, purified water derived by other means of purification could be equally suitable where deionised water is specified.
High purity water	It is prepared in a similar way as deionized water but it is to be used shortly after its production so as to avoid any adventitious contamination that could occour upon storage. It is used as a reagent solvent as well as for cleaning.	It is prepared by distilling previously deionsed water, and then filtering it through a 0.45-µm membrane. This water should have an online conductivity of not more than 0.15 µs/cm at 25°. It may be used where the use of ammonia-free water is specified.
Carbon dioxide-free water	It is produced by vigorous boiling of purified water for at least 5 minutes followed by colling and keeping it protected from absoption of atmospheric carbon dioxide as co2 tends to drive down the water ph. It is used as solvent in ph related or ph sensitive determinations or as a solvent in carbonate sensitive reagents or determinations. It can also be used in optical rotation and color and clarity of solution tests.	This is purified water that has been vigorously boiled for at least 5 minutes, then cooled and protected from absorption of atmospheric carbon dioxide. Most of the uses of this grade of water are either associated as a solvent in ph-related or ph-sensitive reagents or determinations. It is also used in certain optical rotation tests and in the tests for appearance of solution. In addition to boiling, deionization could be an effective process for Removing carbon dioxide.

Alcohol (Ethanol)

Next to water, alcohol is the most useful solvent in pharmacy.

- It is used as a primary solvent for many organic compounds.

- With water it acts as a cosolvent and increases the solubility of drugs. Alcohol is often preferred because of its miscibility with water and its ability to dissolve many water-insoluble ingredients, including drug substances, flavorants, and antimicrobial preservatives.

- Alcohol is frequently used with other solvents, as glycols and glycerin, to reduce the amount of alcohol required.

- It also is used in liquid products as an antimicrobial preservative alone or as a co-preservative with parabens, benzoates, sorbates and other agents.

Disadvantages

It produces pharmacologic and potential toxic effects of alcohol when ingested in pharmaceutical products particularly by children. Hence, it should not be given to children below 6 years. For OTC (over the counter) oral product for children the recommended alcohol-content limit is 0.5 %.

Age of the Child/Adult	Recommended alcohol limit
<6 years	0.5 %
6-12 years	5.0 %
> 12 years and adults	10.0%

Glycerin (Glycerol)

- Glycerin is a clear syrupy liquid with a sweet taste.
- It is miscible both with water an alcohol.
- Glycerin has preservative qualities.

Disadvantages

As a solvent, it is comparable to alcohol, but because of its viscosity, solutes are slowly soluble in it unless it is rendered less viscous by heating.

Propylene Glycol

It is a viscous liquid, is miscible with water and alcohol. It is useful solvent with a wide range of application and is frequently substituted for glycerin in pharmaceutical formulation.

Buffers

A buffer is a compound or mixture of compounds that, by its presence in solution, resists changes in pH upon addition of small quantities of acid or base.

Buffering agents are necessary to resist the change of pH upon dilution or addition of acid or alkali in the liquid preparation.

The usual buffering agents used in oral liquid preparations are *acetate buffer* and *phosphate buffer*.

Buffer	Mixture of	Buffering Range	Chemical formula
Acetate buffer	Glacial acetic acid Potassium, sodium, ammonium salt of acetic acid	pH 2.8 to 6.0	
Phosphate buffer	Potassium dihydrogen phosphate Di-sodium hydrogen phosphate	pH 2.0 to 8.0	

Buffering is required to:

1. Keeping weakly acidic or basic drug in solution
2. Increase the stability of the drug
3. Resist the change of pH upon dilution or addition of acid or alkali (e.g. leaching or alkali from glass container).

Sweeteners

Solutions come in immediate contact with the taste buds (on the tongue). Drugs and other adjuvants are generally not good to taste (i.e. not palatable). To enhance palatability and to mask the taste of the drugs etc. sweeteners are used. Sweeteners can be classified as:

(i) *Natural Sweeteners*: Glucose, Sucrose, Sucralose, Stevia

(ii) *Artificial Sweeteners*: Saccharin, Aspartame.

Sucrose

Source: Commercially sucrose is obtained from sugarcane, beet root and Sorghum.

Advantages

- It is soluble in aqueous medium.
- It is available in highly purified form at reasonable price.
- It is chemically and physically stable in the pH range of 4.0 to 8.0.
- It is frequently used in conjunction with sorbitol, glycerin and other polyols.
- Above 66.7 % w/w concentration, mold growth will not take place.

Disadvantages

Concentration of sucrose solution above 66.7% (w/w) the sucrose crystallize making the solution hazy (i.e. reducing the gloss of the solution).

    Caps of the containers are generally found to be locked due to this crystallization. Sorbitol, glycerin or other polyols are used to reduce the crystallization.

Liquid Glucose

Liquid glucose is an extremely viscid substance that imparts both body (i.e highly viscous) and sweetness to liquid formulations.

    Preparation Partial hydrolysis of starch with strong acid produces liquid glucose. Its main component is dextrose and maltose.

Saccharin (Sodium and Calcium salts are soluble)

Advantages

- Saccharin is used to supplement sugars and polyols as sweeteners.

- It is approximately 250 to 500 times as sweet as sugar.

- It has no calorie value, hence can be given to obese patients and diabetic patients.

Disadvantages: It has a bitter after taste.

Aspartame

Aspartame is the methyl ester of aspartic acid and phenylalanine.

Advantages

- It is approximately 200 times sweeter than sugar.

- No bitter after taste.

- Solubility in water is adequate for formulation purpose.

Disadvantage

Although it is very stable as dry powder, its stability in aqueous solutions is pH and temperature dependent. it is stable at pH between 3.4 and 5.0 and at refrigerated temperature.

COLORANTS

To enhance the appeal of the vehicle, a coloring agent is generally used which matches well with the flavour employed in the preparation e.g. green with mint, brown with chocolate flavor etc. The colorant used is generally water soluble, non-reactive with other components, and color-stable at the pH range.

Under the intensity of light that the liquid preparation is likely to be exposed during its shelf-life.

N.B. From the psychological point of view the scheme may be as follows:

Color:

Red ⟶ ▮ Orange ⟶ ▮ Yellow ⟶ Green ⟶ ▮ Blue ⟶ ▮ Violet

Psychological reactions:

Exciting ⟶ Cheerful ⟶ Tranquilizing ⟶ Subduing

Desirable properties of a coloring agent

1. Must be harmless, should have no physiological activity
2. It should be a definite compound because then its coloring power will be reliable.
3. Its tinctorial (coloring) power should be high so that only small quantities are required.
4. It should be unaffected by light, temperature, micro-organisms, pH changes.
5. It should not interfere with other adjuvants.
6. It must be free from objectionable odour and taste.
7. It must be inexpensive.

Example

- Coal tar colors e.g. Amaranth
- The permitted colors do not always give satisfactory shades when used alone but most popular tints and shades can be obtained by blending

  e.g. Green S and Tartrazine Solution B.P.C. contains Green S (greenish blue) and Tartrazine (Yellow green)

Some FD&C approved colors:

Dye	Shade in Solution	Hue in Powder Form	Common Name(s)	Chemical formula	Solubitlity
FD&C Blue 1	Sky Blue	Greenish Blue	Brilliant Blue FCF	$C_{37}H_{34}N_2Na_2O_9S_3$	Water-soluble
FD&C Blue 2	Deep Blue	Deep Blue	Indigotine, Indigo	$C_{16}H_8N_2Na_2O_8S_2$	Water-soluble
FD&C Red 3	Pink	Bluish Pink	Erythosine	$C_{20}H_6I_4Na_2O_5$	Water-soluble
FD&C Red 40	Brownish Red	Yellowish Red	NT Red, Allura Red AC	$C_{18}H_{14}N_2Na_2O_8S_2$	Water-soluble
FD&C Yellow 5	Bright Yellow	Lemon Yellow	Tartrazine	$C_{16}H_9N_4Na_3O_9S_2$	Water-soluble
FD&C Yellow 6	Orange	Reddish Yellow	Sunset Yellow FCF	$C_{16}H_{10}N_2Na_2O_7S_2$	Water-soluble

PRESERVATIVES

Specific organisms generally recognized as undesirable in oral liquids include *Salmonella* species, *Escherichia coli*, *Enterobacter* species, *Pseudomonas* species (commonly *Pseudomonas aeruginosa*), *Clostridium* and *Candida albicans*.

Source of contamination:

Raw materials, processing containers and equipment, the manufacturing environment, operators, packaging materials and the user.

Characteristics of an ideal preservative

1. It must be effective against a broad spectrum of microorganisms.
2. It must be physically, chemically and microbiologically stable for the lifetime of the product.
3. It must be nontoxic, non-sensitizing, adequately soluble, compatible with other formulation components, and acceptable with respect to taste and odour at the concentrations used.

Some pharmaceutically useful preservative

Class	Preservative	Concentration (%)	Uses
Acidic	Phenol	0.2 - 0.5	Have characteristic odor and unstable when exposed to oxygen, hence used rarely.
	Chlorocresol o-Phenyl phenol Alkyl esters of parahydroxy benzoic acid (e.g. Methyl and Propyl Paraben)	0.05 - 0.1 0.005 - 0.01 0.001 - 0.2	Mostly used, Adequately soluble in water, Have both antifungal and antibacterial activity, Methyl & Propyl ester at a ratio of 10 to 1 produce a synergistic effect
	Benzoic acid and its salts Boric acid and its salts Sorbic acid and its salts	0.1 - .0.3 0.5 - 1.0 0.05 - 0.2	Mostly used, Have antibacterial action and antifungal action, Water soluble.
Neutral	Chlorbutanol Benzyl alcohol β-Phenyl ethyl alcohol	0.5 1.0 0.2 - 1.0	These are volatile alcohols, hence, have odor and loss of preservative action on aging. Not used in oral liquid preparations. Used in ophthalmic, nasal and parenteral products.

Contd....

Class	Preservative	Concentration (%)	Uses
Mercu-rial	Thiomersal Phenyl mercuric acetate and nitrate (PMA & PMN) Nitromersol	0.001 - 0.1 0.002 - 0.005 0.001 - 0.1	Not used in oral liquid preparations. Used in ophthalmic, nasal and parenteral products. *Disadvantage*: Mercurials readily reduced to free mercury.
Quarte-rnary ammo-nium comp-ounds	Benzalkonium chloride Cetylpyridinium chloride	0.004 - 0.02 0.01 - 0.02	Not used in oral preparations. Used in ophthalmic, nasal and parenteral solutions. *Disadvantages*: Inactivated by variety of anionic substances.

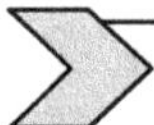

Flavors

An objectionable taste may lead to nausea, vomiting and refusal to take the preparation regularly or not at all. On the other hand, an attractive flavour will encourage continuation of treatment. The four basic taste sensations are salty, bitter, sweet and sour. A combination of flavoring agents is usually required to mask these taste sensations effectively.

Flavor selection

Taste sensation	Recommended flavor
Salty	Butterscotch, maple, apricot, peach, vanilla, wintergreen mint.
Bitter	Wild cherry, walnut, chocolate, mint combinations, anise etc.
Sweet	Fruit and berry, vanilla
Sour	Citrus flavors, liquorice, root beer, raspberry

Flavor adjuncts

Menthol, chloroform and various salts frequently are used as flavor adjuncts and are sometimes referred to as *desensitizing agents*. They impart a flavor and odor of their own to the product and have a mild anaesthetic effect on the sensory receptor organs associated with taste.

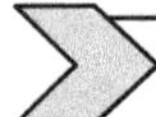

Monophasic Systems

Aromatic waters: According to Indian Pharmacopoeia (I.P., 2018), aromatic waters as clear, saturated aqueous solutions of volatile oils or other aromatic substances. These volatile oils (e.g. Rose oil, peppermint oil, anise oil, spearmint oil etc.), or aromatic substances (e.g. camphor, chloroform etc.) containing saturated solutions are enriched with both the essential oil and the water-soluble volatile components of a plant and thus possesses the taste as that of natural substances. Thus, these are employed as flavored or perfumed vehicles.

Aromatic waters comprise a broader range of both the water and fat-soluble volatile constituents of a plant which contributes to their efficacy and safety. Some of their **advantages** over pure essential oils and tinctures are listed hereunder:

✓ A gentle and balanced action

✓ Offering the essential oil component in an aqueous medium

✓ The convenience of a tincture without the alcohol

✓ A highly convenient preparation

✓ Traditional support for safety and efficacy

Disadvantages:

✓ Deterioration may be due to volatilization, decomposition or mould growth

✓ Becomes cloudy with time due to microbial/fungal growth.

✓ Volatile oils solutions represent an incompatibility problem of salting out. Talc is added as a distributing agent, to increase the saturation/distribution of volatile oil in water and to yield a clear solution by absorbing excess volatile oil.

Broadly aromatic waters can be categorized in *two classes-*

Simple aromatic waters: These encompass purified water as a solvent but do not contain alcohol and are mainly used as vehicles e.g. Chloroform water.

Concentrated aromatic waters: These are alcoholic non aqueous preparations (comprise alcohol as solvent for the volatile constituents) containing 2% of volatile oils and are approximately forty times stronger than the simple aromatic waters. Examples of concentrated aromatic waters are Camphor Water BP, Concentrated Peppermint Water BP, Concentrated Caraway Water BPC, Concentrated Cinnamon Water BPC, Concentrated Dill Water BPC, Concentrated Anise Water BPC etc.

Methods of Preparation

Aromatic waters are prepared employing various techniques, some of which are:

✓ *Solution Process (e.g. Peppermint water):*

Approach-I: The volatile oil is shaken with 500 times its volume of Purified Water IP. The mixture is shaken at intervals for a period of 15 minutes. The mixture is set aside for 12 h or overnight and filtered.

Approach-II: (Using distributing agents): The volatile oil is triturated with a sufficient quantity of powdered talc or kieselghur, or pulped filter paper in a mortar. Purified Water IP 500 times the volume of oil is taken and mixed. Then, the solution is filtered. (*Note-* Talc, kieselghur, pulp of filter paper are called distributing agents. The volatile oils get adsorbed on the particle surface and a large surface area helps in quick dissolution of the oil into water).

✓ ***Dilution from concentrated waters:*** Concentrated aromatic water is prepared as per the formula given in the I.P. One ml of concentrated aromatic water is diluted with 39 ml of Purified Water IP and mixed.

✓ ***Distillation process (e.g. Strong Rose water):*** The drug or essential oil is distilled with water until the specific volume of distillate has been collected. The distillate is shaken thoroughly, allowed to stand for not less than 12 hours and any excess oil is removed.

Therapeutic Use

Aromatic waters such as chamomile, lavender, rose water are utilized as excellent topical preparations for external application due to their wide array of therapeutic actions-soothing, astringent, anti-inflammatory, antiseptic, and cooling actions to the skin and mucus membranes.

Few Examples

Simple Aromatic Water	Concentrated Aromatic Water	Dilution		Use
		Conc. Arom. Water	Purified Water	
Anise Water	Concentrated Anise Water	1ml	39ml	Flavor, Carminative, Mild expectorant
Camphor Water	Concentrated Camphor Water	1ml	39ml	Flavor, Carminative, Mild expectorant, Vehicle, Stimulant
Caraway Water	Concentrated Caraway Water	1ml	39ml	Flavor, Carminative
Chloroform Water	Chloroform Water Double Strength (DS)	1ml	39ml	Preservative, Flavor
Cinnamon Water	Concentrated Cinnamon Water	1ml	39ml	Flavor, Carminative
Dil Water	Concentrated Dil Water	1ml	39ml	Flavor, Carminative (particularly for infants in gripe water)
Peppermint Water	Concentrated Peppermint Water	1ml	39ml	Flavor, Carminative, Weak Preservative
Rose water	Concentrated Rose Water	1ml	39ml	Antioxidant activity
Hamamelis water	Concentrated Hammamelis Water	1ml	39ml	Rub, perfume and as an astringent in after-shave lotions

Dose: Usually 15-30 ml (simple aromatic waters)

Varies (Concentrated aromatic waters)

Shelf Life: Most waters have shelf life of 6-8 months.

Storage: Should be stored in air tight, amber-colored glass bottles in cool place (to prevent from intense heat and light)

Caution: Label should bear in red ink.

(i) 'Protect it from direct exposure to sun light'. In case of chloroform water-Use fresh preparation as chloroform gets converted to poisonous phosgene gas with passage of time.

(ii) Do not use if preparation becomes cloudy in appearance.

Commercial Formulations

Active Ingredient(s)	Marketed Preparation (Manufacturer)
Rose Water	Gulabari (Dabur Pvt. Ltd)
Dill Water	Woodward's gripe water (TTK Healthcare Ltd.)

Practicals Based on Aromatic Waters

1. AIM- To prepare Chloroform Water I.P. (40 ml)

Ingredients	Qty. prescribed	Qty. used
Chloroform	2.5 ml.	0.1ml
Purified Water q.s.	1000.0 ml	40ml

Apparatus: Glass beaker, measuring cylinder and volumetric pipette

Theory: Aromatic waters are clear, saturated aqueous solution of volatile compounds. They are generally prepared by simple dilution or distillation method and usually have the taste and smell of the corresponding aromatic substance. Chloroform ($CHCl_3$) is a clear colorless liquid having specific gravity 1.474 to 1.479 and possesses characteristic odor with burning sweet taste. The solubility of chloroform is 1 in 800 parts of water. Chloroform water is prepared by simply dissolving chloroform in vehicle viz. water with continuous vigorous shaking till both the liquids form a homogenous solution. As both the liquids are miscible with each other at the prescribed concentration, the solution formed is clear. Aromatic waters do not contain any added preservative. Hence, they are prepared under hygienic conditions. They are meant for consumption within 5-7 days after opening the bottle. Therefore, the label should clearly mention "Discard if the contents appear cloudy" meaning that the preparation should not be consumed as it may have become contaminated with fungus if the bottle had been kept for many days after opening.

Procedure: Measure 0.1ml of chloroform. Take about 10ml of water and dissolve chloroform in water with continuous shaking. Then make up the volume by adding sufficient purified water (40ml) and dispense it.

Storage: Store at cool and dry place away from direct heat and light.

Uses: Preservative vehicle for liquid preparations.

Specimen Label: The specimen label for Chloroform Water IP is given as:

<table>
<tr><td colspan="3" align="center">CHLOROFORM WATER (I.P) 40 ml</td></tr>
<tr>
<td>Composition:
Each 40 ml contains,
Chloroform- 0.1 ml
Purified water q.s.- 40 ml
Dose: 15 to 30 ml
Storage: Store in airtight,
light-resistant container
in cool place.</td>
<td>AQUACHLOR®
(Aromatic Water)
(Used for perfuming,
flavoring the formulation,
as vehicle and also as a
preservative at 25% v/v)

PROTECT FROM SUN
LIGHT
NOT FOR INJECTION</td>
<td>Mfg. Lic. No.- AKT/2018
Batch No.- HG 4311
Mfg. Date- Mar. 2018
Exp. Date- Feb. 2019
M.R.P.- Rs. 39.00
(Inclusive of all taxes)
Mfd. By: AKT PHARMA
SADIQ ROAD, PATIALA
PB-147002</td>
</tr>
</table>

2. AIM- To prepare Camphor Water I.P. (40ml)

Ingredients	Qty. prescribed	Qty. used
Camphor	1.0 g	40mg
Alcohol 90% v/v	20.0 ml.	0.8ml
P. water q.s.	1000.0 ml.	40ml

Apparatus Required: Glass beaker, measuring cylinder and volumetric pipette

Theory: Camphor $[C_{10}H_{16}O]$ is a ketone or a keto-tetrahydro-cymene, obtained from *Cinnamomum camphora*. Camphor occurs as a colorless, transparent, crystalline solid. It has a powerful penetrating odor, and pungent, somewhat bitter, taste, followed by a slight sensation of cold. It has specific gravity 0.986 to 0.996. Synthetic camphor differs from the natural camphor in being optically inactive instead of dextrorotatory. Camphor is readily soluble in alcohol (1 in 1.25). Camphor water is prepared by dissolving camphor in purified water using alcohol as cosolvent. Since camphor is insoluble in water, so it is firstly dissolved in alcohol. Then purified water is added to alcoholic solution water drop wise with continuous stirring.

Procedure: Weight 0.04g of camphor and dissolve in 0.08ml of 90% v/v alcohol. Now add water to alcoholic solution in successive portions to purified water. Shake well after each addition.

Category: Pharmaceutical aid.

Dose: 30 to 60 ml.

Storage: Store at cool and dry place away from direct heat and light.

Uses: Carminative and Flavoring vehicle.

Specimen Label: The specimen label for Camphor Water IP is given as:

CAMPHOR WATER (I.P) 40 ml		
Composition: Each 40 ml contains- Camphor- 0.04 g Ethanol (90%)- 0.08 ml Purified water q.s.- 40 ml **Dose:** 30 to 60 ml. **Storage:** Store in airtight, light-resistant container in cool place.	**AQUAPHOR®** (Aromatic Water) (Flavoring agent, Mild carminative, Diaphoretic and Expectorant) PROTECT FROM SUN LIGHT NOT FOR INJECTION	Mfg. Lic. No.- HG/2018 Batch No.- AKT 4311 Mfg. Date- Nov. 2018 Exp. Date- Sep. 2019 M.R.P.- Rs. 60.00 (Inclusive of all taxes) Mfd. By: AKT PHARMA SADIQ ROAD, PATIALA PB-147002

3. AIM- To prepare Concentrated Peppermint Water B.P. (40ml.)

Ingredients	Qty prescribed	Qty prescribed
Peppermint oil	20.0 ml	0.8ml
Alcohol 90% v/v	600.0 ml	24ml
Purified water q.s.	1000.0 ml	40ml

Theory: Concentrated aromatic waters are 40-fold more concentrated than simple aromatic waters. One part of concentrated aromatic water should be diluted with 39 parts of water to produce simple aromatic water. Peppermint oil is extracted from *Mentha piperita* (Family- *Labiatae*). The main chemical components of peppermint oil are menthol, menthone, 1,8-cineole. Peppermint oil is non-toxic and non-irritant in low dilutions, but sensitization may be a problem due to the menthol content. It can cause irritation to the skin and mucus membranes and should be kept well away from the eyes. Peppermint oil should be stored in closed containers kept in a dry place, avoiding sunshine and rain. Peppermint water is prepared by using a distributing agent such as talc. Measured amount of oil is dissolved in alcohol and the alcoholic mixture is dissolved in sufficient volume of water till it solubilizes. Then talc (5g per 100ml of preparation) is added to adsorb excess of oil which remain suspended in the solution and thus provide a clean, uniform and homogeneous formulation. The precipitated talc is filtered off. (**Note-** The talc used should be sterilized because it contains high content of *Clostridium* which is causative agent of tetanus).

Procedure: Dissolve peppermint oil in 90% v/v alcohol and add sufficient purified water in successive small quantities to produce 40ml. Shake it vigorously after each addition and then add 5g of talc per 100ml and allow to rest for four hours finally, filter the solution. Filter again until clear solution is obtained.

Storage: Keep in cool and dry place away from direct sunlight.

Uses: Flavoring agent, Carminative, Weak preservative, Vehicle soluble

Specimen Label: The specimen label for Peppermint Water BP is given as:

PEPPERMINT WATER (B.P) 40 ml		
Composition: **Each 50 ml contains:** Oil of peppermint- 0.1 ml Distilled water q.s.- 50 ml **Dose:** 10 to 40 ml **Storage:** Store in well-closed, light-resistant container cool place to volatilization of oil.	**AQUAMINT®** (Aromatic Water) (Used as an antispasmodic and carminative in flatulence of the gastrointestinal tract, cramping and bloating, flatulent colic to relieve nausea and vomiting, and as a gentle aromatic stimulant) PROTECT FROM SUN LIGHT NOT FOR INJECTION	Mfg. Lic. No.- HAT/2018 Batch No.- AKH 4311 Mfg. Date- Jan. 2018 Exp. Date- Dec. 2019 M.R.P.- Rs. 49.00 (Inclusive of all taxes) Mfd. By: AKT PHARMA SADIQ ROAD, PATIALA PB-147002

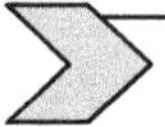

Syrups

Syrups are concentrated aqueous preparations (saturated solutions) of sugar or sugar-substitute in purified water with or without added flavoring agents and medicinal substances. These preparations contain 66.7%w/w (as per I.P or B.P.) or 85%w/v (as per U.S.P) concentration of sugar which resist bacterial growth by virtue of their exosmotic effect on micro-organisms. Syrups that contain less than 85% sucrose, a sufficient concentration of polyol (e.g. sorbitol, glycerin, propylene glycol or polyethylene glycol) should be added to have the required osmotic pressure.

Crucial components:

✓ **Sugar or its substitute** e.g. sucrose or dextrose; *sugar subsitutes-* sorbitol, *glycerin, propylene glycol.* Methyl cellulose or hydroxyethyl cellulose are also used assyrup-like vehicles (directly absorbs to blood without hydrolyzation).

✓ **Antimicrobial preservative-** e.g. 67.7%w/w of sucrose acts as self-preservative due to high osmotic pressure. If needed 5-10% ethanol may be added as preservative and to increase the solubility of sucrose. In some dilute preparations- benzoic acid, sodium benzoate, methyl paraben may be used as preservative.

✓ **Flavoring agents-**e.g. *Tinctures:* L emon tincture, ginger tincture. *Fruit juices-* Raspberry, Wild cherry, *Essence-*Vanilla, Cocoa and Orange.

✓ **Taste maskers/enhancers-**Although when syrup is ingested, only a fraction of dissolved drug actually makes contact with the taste buds, yet the remainder of the drug being carried past them and down the throat in the containment of the viscous syrup. But, antitussive syrups (e.g. linctus) the thick sweet syrup provides soothing effect on the irritated tissues of the throat as it passes over them. In preparations containing bitter drugs, some taste enhancers or taste masking agents are also used apart from flavoring agents e.g. citric acid.

✓ **Stablizers/Adjunts-** e.g. Na-EDTA, Glycerin, sorbitol or propylene glycol are employed to prevent crystallization. Tween 80 may be added to dissolve certain insoluble substances and thus produce clear syrup.

✓ **Coloring agent-**e.g. Amaranth (pink red), Compound Tartrazine (yellow), Green S with Tartrazine (Green).

✓ **Vehicles-**e.g. Purified water

CLASSIFICATION OF SYRUPS

➢ *Simple Syrup:* Encompasses only sucrose and purified water e.g. Syrup USP

➢ *Medicated syrup:* Encompasses medicinal substances e.g. Chlorpheniramine maleate syrup, Ipecac syrup, Chloral hydrate syrup.

➢ *Non-medicated or Flavored syrup:* Encompasses flavoring vehicles, used for flavoring a liquid oral preparation e.g. Cherry Syrup, Cocoa Syrup, Orange syrup, Raspberry Syrup.

Storage conditions: Place in cool place and store it in tight, narrow mouthed, amber color or plain bottle.

Self- preservatory nature of syrup: Although, simple syrup NF comprises of saturated solutions of 85% w/v sucrose. However, the self preservatory action of syrup is not due to high concentration of sucrose, but due to unavailability of water required for the growth of micro-organisms. Let's understand it:

85% w/v syrup has a specific gravity of 1.313

i.e. 100 ml syrup contains 85 gm sucrose

Weight of 100 ml syrup = 100 x 1.313 = 131.3 gm

∴ Weight of water present in 100 ml syrup = (131.3 − 85) gm= 46.3 gm

Volume of water present in 100 ml syrup = 46.3 ml

∴ Volume of sucrose present in 100 ml syrup= (100 − 46.3) ml= 53.7 ml

∴ 100 ml 85% syrup contains

Ingredients	Weight	Volume
Sugar	85.0 g	53.7 ml
Water	46.3 g	46.3 ml
Syrup (total)	131.3 g	100.0 ml

The solubility of sucrose in water is 1 g in 0.5 ml

∴To dissolve 85 g sugar required will be = 85 x 0.5 ml

$$= 42.5 \text{ ml}$$

Thus, only a very slight excess of water (46.3 − 42.5 = 3.8 ml per 100 ml of syrup) is employed in the preparation of syrup. The sight excess of water permits the syrup to remain physically stable under conditions of varying temperature.

Method of Formulation: Some of the techniques employed are mentioned hereunder:

✓ Heat based approach

✓ Non-heat based or cold approach

✓ Using percolation

Heat based Approaches:

Sugar and some heat stable components are added to the purified water, and heat is applied (to facilitate the rapid solution of sugar) until hot syrup is formed. The mixture is then allowed to cool, and the final volume is made up by adding water.

Excessive heating results in hydrolyzation into dextrose (D-glucose), and fructose (levulose), the combination is called as invert sugar whereas the process is termed as inversion reaction.

In such processes, some of the inversion cannot be avoided however; the speed or reaction can be enhanced by the presence of acids, the hydrogen ion acting as a catalyst to reaction.

Advantages:

Invert sugar is colorless and sweeter than sucrose.

Disadvantages:

Syrup darkens due to the effect of heat on the levulose portion of invert sugar

Overheading of syrup leads to caramelization of the sucrose (ambered coloured byproduct) and becomes susceptible to fermentation and microbial growth.

Syrups cannot be sterilized by autoclaving owing to degradation.

Cold Process (Non-heatbased approaches)

Sucrose and some other agents are dissolved in large vessel containing purified water followed by thorough agitation of the mixture. Tinctures and extracts are directly used as active ingredient in the formulation of syrup if the excipients are water soluble only. However, if the extract contains alcohol soluble excipients then the sucrose is directly added for mixing.

Percolation

Purified water or an aqueous solution is passed slowly through a bed of crystalline sucrose, thus dissolving it and forming the syrup. If required, a portion of the percolate is recycled again.

Commercial Examples

Medicated Syrup:

Syrup	Drug	Commercial Product	Uses
Bronchodilator	Albuterol Sulphate	Ventolin (Glaxosmithkline)	Relief of bronchospasm of obstruction airway disease
Hemostatic	Aminoaproic acid	Amicar (Xanodyne)	Urinary fibrinolysis
Antiviral	Amantadine HCl	Symmetral (Allaince)	Idiopathic parkinsons disease and Relief from A2 viral strains
Anticonvulsant	Sodium valproate	Depkene (Abbot)	Adjunt therapy in simple, compex and partial seizure therapy
Analgesic	Paracetamol	Progesic (FT metiska Farma)	For fever
Anticholinergic	Diclomine HCl	Bentyl (Axcam Scandipharm)	Treatment of peptic ulcer

Non-Medicated or Flavored Syrup:

Syrup	Ingredient	Use
Cocoa Syrup	Cocoa powder, sugar, water	As flavoring agent
Raspberry Syrup	Raspberry	As flavoring agent
Orange Syrup	Orange, water	As flavoring agent
Corn Syrup	glucose, maltose and higher oligosaccharides	As food additive
Glucose Syrup	Dextrose, maltose and higher sachharides	As vehicle, sweetener
Maple syrup	Sucrose, water, monosaccharides, glucose and fructose	As sweetener
Cane syrup	Sugar cane juice	As sweetener
Golden syrup	Water, sugar and citric acid	As sweetener

Practicals Based on Syrups

1. AIM: To prepare a simple syrup I.P./B.P.(50 g)

Ingredients	Qty. prescribed (1000 g)	Qty. used (50 g)
Sucrose	667.00 g	33.3 g
Purified water q.s.	1000.00 g	Vol. up to 50.0 g

Theory: Syrup are saturated solution of sucrose in water containing exactly 66.7% w/w of sucrose according to I.P. and 85% w/v of sucrose according to U.S.P. Syrups are highly viscous and sweet in nature. Therefore, they are used in many pharmaceutical preparations as vehicles for pediatric purposes and for masking the bitter taste of drugs. They are also used as binders in tablet granules, bulk former in sugar coated tablets, coating for chewable tablets etc. Simple syrup needs to be carefully prepared because if the concentration of sucrose in preparation is less than 66.7% w/w then bacterial growth will take place and if more than 66.7% w/w then sucrose will crystallize. Many times syrups may contain polyols like glycerol, propylene glycol, polyethylene glycol for preventing crystallization of sucrose especially when more than 66.7% w/w sucrose has been used.

Method of Preparation (Gravimetric): Tare an empty beaker and note down its weight. Weigh 33.3 g of sucrose and place it in the tared beaker. Add little quantity of water to this sucrose and heat on water bath with occasional stirring until it dissolves. Tare the beaker after wiping the exterior surface to remove water. Add sufficient water or evaporate the excess water to obtain a weight equal to weight of the empty beaker plus 50g.

Storage: Keep it in a cool place.

Uses:

✓ As a pharmaceutical aid.

✓ As a sweetener in chewable tablets and liquid preparations.

✓ As taste enhancers or taste maskers and providing stability in coating of tablets.

✓ As a suspending agent prevents setting of particles.

✓ As drug delivery vehicles for pediatric solutions.

Specimen Label: The specimen label for simple syrup I.P. is given as:

SIMPLE SYRUP (I.P.) 50 g		
Composition: **Each 50g contains:** Sucrose- 33.3 g Distilled water- q.s. 50 g **Dose:** 10 to 40 ml **Storage:** Store in a cool and dry place. **Precautions:** NOT FOR DIABETIC PATIENTS.	SIMROF® Oral Solution (Used as a sweetener and as a vehicle) PROTECT FROM SUN LIGHT NOT FOR INJECTION	Mfg. Lic. No.- HAT/2018 Batch No.- AKH 4311 Mfg. Date- Jan. 2018 Exp. Date- Dec. 2019 M.R.P.- Rs. 49.00 (Inclusive of all taxes) Mfd. By: AKT PHARMA SADIQ ROAD, PATIALA PB-147002

2.   AIM- To prepare invert Syrup I.P. (30 g)

Ingredients	Qty prescribed	Qty. used
Sucrose	667.00 g	22.2 g
Purified water q.s.	1000.00 g	30.00 g

Note: Small amount of HCl and NaHCO₃*

Theory- Syrups are saturated solution of sucrose in water containing precisely about 66.7% w/w of sucrose according to I.P. They are highly viscous, sweet and stable pharmaceutical preparations. Invert syrup which is prepared by treating simple syrup with dil. HCl results in hydrolysis of sucrose, forming one molecule each of glucose and fructose. Invert syrup can also be prepared by using invertase enzyme. Fructose being sweeter than glucose and sucrose results in enhanced sweetness of the formulation.

Advantages: Invert syrup has following advantages:

1.   It is sweeter than simple syrup due to formation of dextro- and levo rotating sugars namely glucose and fructose respectively.

2.   Darker in color hence addition of extra color can be avoided.

3.   Does not crystallize quickly i.e. more stable and hence is added to simple syrup to prevent its crystallization.

Procedure: Prepare Simple syrup as described in the earlier experiment. Then add few drops of hydrochloric acid until the pH reaches 4. Check with the help of pH paper. Then drop wise add sodium bicarbonate solution till the pH reaches 7. Finally, dispense the formulation. Sodium bicarbonate is used for neutralizing the excess acid.

Uses: Pharmaceutical aid.

3.   AIM- To prepare Compound syrup of Ferrous Phosphate BPC'68 (30 ml) (Synonym- Perrish's Food, Perrish Syrup, Chemical Food)

Ingredients	Qty. (1000 ml)	Qty. (30 ml)
Iron (Ferrous protosulphate)	4.3 g	129 g
Phosphoric acid	48 ml	1.44 ml
Calcium Carbonate	3.6 g	108 mg
Potassium bicarbonate	1g	30 mg
Sodium Phosphate	1g	30 mg
Cochineal	3.5 g	105 mg
Sucrose	700 g	21 gm
Orange flavor (Orange- Flower water of commerce)	50 ml	1.5 ml
Purified water qs.	1000 ml	30 ml

Theory: The compound syrup of iron phosphate or (known as *Syrupus Ferri Phosphatis Compositus*), (was listed in B.P.C. 1968 edition) is also called

Parrish's Syrup or Chemical food. It is useful tonic especially for children. It is administered in doses of 0.5-2.0 drahms (or 1.84- 7.4 ml) in conjuction with cod liver oil.

Method of Preparation (Volumetric):

Dilute 20ml of the phosphoric acid with 25 ml of water, add the iron and heat gently on a water-bath until the iron has dissolved. Add the solution to the calcium carbonate, the potassium bicarbonate and the sodium phosphate, previously triturated with the remainder of the phosphoric acid and 80 ml of water. Boil the cochineal with 375ml of water for 15 minutes, cool, strain, and pass sufficient water through the strainer to produce 800 ml. Filter the iron solution into the syrup thus obtained. Add the orange flower water, pass sufficient water through the filter to produce the required volume, mix, allow to stand for at least 8 hours, and filter if necessary. Pack and label the preparation.

Uses: Used as tonic for the growth of body, bone and muscles.

Dosage: One desert spoonful to be taken three times daily.

Commercial Examples: Marketed under trade name as *Eastern's Syrup* in early ninetees. Not in use. It was banned due to reports of arsenic in the formulations.

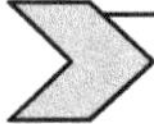

Elixirs

USP XVII defines elixirs *(synonym- Elix.)* are clear, sweet-flavored hydroalcoholic (with alcohol content vary from 5-40% or 10-80 degrees proof) solutions intended for oral medicinal use and are usually flavored to enhance their palatability without affecting the active ingredient. *(*Note: Elixirs were included in I.P. 66 but presently, no longer a part of Indian Pharmacopoeia 2018 except USP or BP)*

Elixir Preparation	Uses	Reference in I.P. 66 (Page No.)
Elixir of Vitriol IP	Pharmaceutical aid	726
Piperazine Citrate Elixir IP	Anthelmintic	568
Simple Elixir IP	Pharmaceutical aid	656
Terpin hydrate Elixir IP	Expectorant	736

Why Elixirs?

✓ For hydrophobic drugs where syrups and suspensions are of no use

✓ For dissolving non- polar compounds

✓ Taste masking aid

Crucial Components of Elixir

1. *Alcohol and Purified Water (Primary Solvents):* Water to Alcohol ratio: the

proportion of alcohol in elixir varies as the different components present in elixir (according to their solubilities). Each elixir requires a specific blend to maintain all the components in solution form. Therefore, elixirs with high alcoholic content contain poorly water-soluble compounds.

2. *Sweeteners:* Agents such as plain and flavored sucrose syrup, glycerol, sorbitol, invert syrup and saccharin sodium are used.

3. *Gycerin and Propylene Glycol (as Visocity builders/stablizers/Adjuncts:* Some compounds are employed to make the elixir stable. e.g. Citirc acid (In neomycin elixir, citric acid is used to adjust pH 4.0 to 5.0 to minimize the darkening that occurs on storage), disodium edetate (to sequester heavy metals that catalyse decomposition of the antibiotics).

4. *Flavorants and Colorants:* Some compounds are used to mask the bitter taste or sourness of drugs flavors-fruit flavor: Blackcurrant syrup (to mask bitter taste of drug), Raspberry Syrup (to mask bitter taste of drug), Compound Orange Syrup (to mask sour and bitter taste of drugs). Many elixirs are attractively colored by coal tar dyes. e.g. Amaranth (magenta red), Compound Tartrazine (saffron), Green S and Tartrazine (Green).

5. *Preservatives:* Vehicles containing 20% v/v alcohol, propylene glycol or glycerol have preservative action. However, benzoic acid, methyl parahydroxybenzoate acid (methyl paraben) or propyl parahydroxynenzoate (propyl paraben) may also be used as additional preservatives.

Classification of Elixirs

1. **Medicated Elixir-** Elixirs containing therapeutically active compounds are known as medicated elixirs Examples- *Antihistamine elixir-* Diphenhydramine HCl, Chlorpheniramine maleate elixir; *Analgesic elixir-* Acetaminophin; *Cardiotonic elixir-* Digoxin; *Antispasmodic elixir-* Hyoscamin sulfate; *Sedative elixir-* Phenobarbital sodium; *Expectorant elixir-*Terpin hydrate.

2. **Non-medicated Elixir:** They are used purely as diluting agents or solvents for drugs containing approximately 25% alcohol. e.g. Simple elixir, Aromatic elixirs-perfumes, Iso-alcoholic elixir or Low alcohol elixir (containing 8-10% v/v alcohol), High alcoholic elixir (containing 75-78% v/v alcohol), Compound benzaldehyde elixir.

   (*Note: Dry Elixirs-* Kim and co-workers has developed the concept of dry elixirs to improve solubility, dissolution and bioavailability of the drug. In dry elixirs, NSAIDs and ethanol were encapsulated in dextrins which enhanced the dissolution and bioabvailability of the drug)

Methods of Preparation:

1. Simple Solution Methods

2. Admixing two or more liquids

In general, elixirs are prepared by dissolving the ingredients with agitation or by admixture of two or more liquid components in the suitable solvent. Usually, the alcohol soluble substances are dissolved in alcohol and water soluble in water separately. As a rule, the aqueous solution is always added to alcoholic solution with constant stirring and the volume is made up with the solvent or vehicle specified in the formulation. At this stage the product may not be clear due to the separation of some of the flavouring agents because the alcoholic strength is reduced. In such case the elixir is allowed to stand for some time to ensure the saturation of the hydroalcoholic solvent and permit the oil globules to coalesce. Talc (~3%) is used to absorb the excess of oils and assist in their removal from solution. Filtration gives a bright clear product.

Commercial Products

Elixir	Drug	Commercial Product	Use
Adrenocortical steroid	Dexamethosone	Dexamethosone elixir (Qualitest)	For allergies, antiinflammtory and skin diseases
Analgesic	Acetaminophen	Children Tylenol elixir (McNeil)	For pain and fever and for patients sensitive to aspirin
Cardiotonic	Digoxin	Lanoxin pediatric elixir (Glaxowellcome)	For myocardial infarction, CCF, atrial fibrillation and other cardiac conditions
Sedatives/Hyp notics	Phenobarbital	Phenobarbital Elixir (Qualitest)	Used as sedative and hypnotic (contain 14% alcohol)

Advantages

✓ Act as self-preservative due to 10-20% alcohol
✓ Provide better stability and maintain balance of the solubility of both water soluble and insoluble substances
✓ Ease to prepare
✓ Act as vehicle
✓ Used as dilution for medicated elixirs
✓ Useful for patients which are unable to swallow the solid dosage forms

Disadvantages:

✓ Less effective than syrups in taste masking of drugs
✓ Cannot be given to children due to high alcoholic content
✓ Contain volatile substances, require air tight storage conditions
✓ Need safe handling due to inflammablilty of the components

Storage: At room temperature (<30°C) in tight, light resistant (protection from direct sunlight) containers.

Practicals based on Elixirs

1. AIM-To prepare Piperazine citrate elixir

Ingredients	Qty. Prescribed (1000 mL)	Qty. (50 mL)
Piperazine citrate	180g	9g
Chloroform Spirit	5ml	0.25 mL
Glycerin	100ml	0.5 mL
Orange Oil	0.25ml	0.0125 mL
Syrup	500ml	25 mL
Purified water qs.	1000ml	50 mL

Theory:

Methods of Preparation:

Weigh 9.0 g of Piperazine citrate and dissolve it in small amount of purified water. Add prescribed amount of orange oil, glycerin, syrup and chloroform spirit in it respectively and mix it vigrously. Sufficient volume of purified water is added to produce the final volume.

Dose: One teaspoonful to be given at night

Storage: Well closed air tight glass containers having screw cap at cool place with protection from sunlight.

Use: Anthelmintic (For the treatment of pinworm, threadworm and roundworm infections)

Specimen Label: The specimen label for **Piperazine citrate elixir BP** is given as:

Piperazine Citrate Elixir BP 50mL		
Composition: **Each 5mL contains:** Piperazine Citrate BP- 900 mg Chloroform Spirit, Orange oil, Syrup, Glycerin and Distilled water q.s.- 50 ml **Dosage:** One teaspoon at night **CAUTION:** Do not exceed the stated dose. If symptoms persist, consult your doctor.	PIPERACIT® (Piperazine Citrate Elixir BP) (For the treatment of pinworm, threadworm and roundworm infections) Keep the container tightly closed Protect from direct sun light KEEP OUT OF THE REACH OF CHILDREN	Mfg. Lic. No.- MPL/42671 Batch No.- KAT 13411 Mfg. Date- May. 2018 Exp. Date- June. 2019 M.R.P.- Rs. 99.00 (Inclusive of all taxes) Mfd. By: COX PHARMA SADIQ ROAD, PATIALA PB-147002

2.   AIM-To prepare paracetamol pediatric elixir BP.

Ingredients	Qty. Prescribed (1000 mL)	Qty. (50 mL)
Paracetamol	24 g	1.2g
Ethanol (96%)	100 ml	5 ml
Propylene glycol	100 ml	5 ml
Concentrated raspberry juice	25 ml	1.25 ml
Chloroform spirit	20 ml	1 ml
Invert syrup	275 ml	13.75 ml
Amaranth solution	2 ml	0.1 ml
Glycerin, qs.	1000.0 ml	50 ml (qs)

Theory: Paediatric paracetamol oral solution is a solution containing 2.4 % w/v of paracetamol in a suitable flavoured vehicle.

Procedure: Mix 5.0 ml of ethanol (96%), with 5.0 ml of propylene glycol and 1.0 ml of chloroform spirit and make a mixture. Weigh 1.2 g of paracetamol powder (solubility of paracetamol is 1 in 79 parts of water, 1 in 20 parts of boiling water) and dissolve it in the resultant mixture and shake it continously, add other additives (such as raspberry juice, amaranth solution and invert syrup- by hydrolyzing 66.7 % solution of sucrose with suitable mineral acid, and neutralising the solution with sodium carbonate) and sufficient amount of glycerin to produce 50 ml.

Uses: As analgesic and antipyretic.

Specimen Label: The specimen label for **Paracetamol pediatric elixir BP**. is given as:

Paracetamol pediatric elixir BP 50mL		
Composition: **Each 5mL contains:** Paracetamol BP- 120 mg Propylene Glycol, Concenterated Respbery Juice, Invert syrup, Amaranth (E123), Glycerol (E422) Ethanol (10% v/v) and Distilled water q.s.- 50 ml **Dosage: FOR CHILDREN** 1-6 YEARS: One to two 5ml teaspoons every 4-6 hours. 3 MONTHS- 1 YEAR: Half to one 5ml teaspoon every 4-6 hours. UNDER 3 MONTHS: On doctor's advice only.	**PARAGESIC®** (Paracetamol Pediatric Elixir BP) (For relief of pain and feverish conditions in children) KEEP THE CONTAINER TIGHTLY CLOSED PROTECT FROM DIRECT SUN LIGHT KEEP OUT OF THE REACH OF CHILDREN **CONTAINS** **PARACETAMOL** Do not give it with any other pacetamol products. Seek medical advice in case of overdose, even if child	Mfg. Lic. No.- PL/42671 Batch No.- HAKT78811 Mfg. Date- Jan. 2022 Exp. Date- Dec. 2023 M.R.P.- Rs. 49.00 (Inclusive of all taxes) Mfd. By: COX PHARMA SADIQ ROAD, PATIALA PB-147002

Contd....

CAUTION: Not more than 4 doses in any 24-hour period. Do not exceed the stated dose. If symptoms 3persist, consult your doctor.	seems well, because of risk of delayed, serious liver damage.	

3. AIM: To prepare streptomycin elixir pediatric BP 1988 (Synonym: Streptomycin mixture, pediatric)

Ingredients	Qty. (1000 ml)	Qty. (40 ml)
Sucrose	750 g	30 g
Streptomycin sulphate	31.4 g	1.25 g
Sodium citrate	9.0 g	360 mg
Methyl hydroxyl benzoate	1.3 g	52 mg
Citric acid	1.0 g	40 mg
Amaranth solution	2 ml	80 mg
Purified water qs.	1000 ml	40 ml

Method of Preparation: Dissolve the methylhydroxybenzoate in 100 ml of water with the aid of gentle heat. Dissolve the sodium citrate, the citric acid and sucrose in the hot solution and cool. Dissolve the streptomycin sulphate in 100 ml of cold water, and mix the two solutions. Add the amaranth solution and sufficient water to produce the required volume and mix.

Dosage: One desert spoonful *t.d.s.*

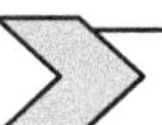

Liniments

Liniments are the viscous, non-aqueous, semi-fluid mixtures (comprise of alcoholic solutions of soap or oily solutions or emulsions) of various medicinal compounds intended for only external application (applied on unbroken skin with or without friction). Most of the formulations are rubbed and massaged onto the affected area and the phenomenon is called as embrocation. In these formulations, alcohol or hydroalcoholic vehicle assists in penetrating the drug into the skin whereas the preparations containing fixed oil or combination of fixed and volatile oil as vehicle helps in spreading and ease of application of the liniment on to the skin. The selection of vehicle for a liniment is based on the solubility of the desired components in various solvents and the type of action desired as mentioned hereunder:

✓ Analgesic (reduces pain),

✓ Astringent (contracts body tissues and reduces permeability of skin)

✓ Antipruritic (reduces itching)

✓ Emollient (Softens dry skin)

✓ Rubefacient (produce local reddening of skin when rubbed, as they increase blood supply to the skin)

✓ Counter irritant (counters strong irritation)

✓ Stimulant (massaged with friction)

It is noted that liniments *should not be applied on bruises or broken skin* as it leads to excessive irritation. These preparations must never be taken internally.

Types: These preparations can be broadly classified into two types:

1. *Alcoholic liniments:* Such preparations penetrate the skin more readily than the oily solutions and generally produce actions like rubefacient, mild counterirritant, mild astringent etc. e.g. Aconite Liniment BPC

2. *Oleogenous liniments:* Such preparations are more useful when applied on the area with massage and provide milder action without irritation. These formulations act solely as protective coatings on the skin. E.g. Methyl salicylate liniment BPC, Turpentine liniment BP

Labelling directions:

✓ For external application only

✓ Shake the bottle well before use

✓ Not to be applied to open wound or broken skin

✓ Prevent any direct contact with eyes

Storage: Such preparations are stored in colored fluted bottle (to indicate an external preparation), well-closed air tight container. It must be stored in a cool place, because it contains volatile ingredients.

Commercial Examples:

Liniment Ingredients	Trade name	Company	Uses
Menthol and oil of wintergreen	Tiger Balm®	Haw Par Healthcare Limited, Singapore	Headache, Joint Pain, Neck and Shoulder Pain
Camphor, Eucaptus oil, Menthol, Nutmeg oil, petrolatum	Vicks Vapo-rub®	Proctor and Gamble, India	cough and congestion
Iodine, Methyl Salicylate, Oleid acid, Paraffin, Petrolatum	Iodex®	GSK, India	Local aches and pains
Thymol, Camphor, Winter Green Oil, Turptentine Oil	Macadex®	Doshi Labratories, Mumbai, india	Lumbago, Sciatica, Muscular Pains, Stiffness of Joints, Neuralgia and sprains

Practicals Based on Liniments

1. AIM- To prepare Camphor Liniment I.P. (20g)

Ingredients	Qty. prescribed (1000 g)	Qty. (20 g)
Camphor	200g	4.0 g
Arachis oil	800g	16 g

Theory- Liniments are the medicated topical solutions or mixture of substances in oil or alcohol meant for application to the unbroken skin with friction. They are typically used to relieve pain and stiffness from sore muscles. They contain volatile ingredient which on exposure to atmosphere evaporates providing a cool effect because of which blood vessel dilates, more blood flows at the applied area and more drug is absorbed into the skin.

Procedure: Place the arachis oil (~16 g) into a suitable dry flask or bottle, heat on a steam bath, add camphor and tighten the container securely with stopper. Agitate to dissolve the camphor (~4 g) without further heating. (*Note:* The liniment should never be prepared in an open dish, as most of the camphor will volatilize. Although "camphorated oil" is often applied to this liniment and also frequently to indicate "Camphor Injection" a sterile 10% solution of camphor in olive oil or other fixed oil and which is used hypodermically as a stimulant. The two products must not be confused).

Uses: Local Analgesic, Rubefacient

Precautions:

Prevent contact with eyes.

Do not apply on broken skin.

For external use only

Specimen Label: The specimen label for Camphor Liniment I.P. (20g) is given as:

<table>
<tr><td colspan="3" align="center">Camphor Liniment I.P. 20 g</td></tr>
<tr>
<td valign="top">Composition:

Each 5 g contains:
Camphor- 1000 mg
Arachis oil qs

Directions:
Apply to affected areas and massage gently 2 or 3 times a day until the condition is relieved.</td>
<td valign="top" align="center">CAMLIN®
(For relief of aches, pain and sprains)
KEEP THE CONTAINER TIGHTLY CLOSED
FOR EXTERNAL USE ONLY
KEEP OUT OF THE REACH OF CHILDREN</td>
<td valign="top" align="center">Mfg. Lic. No.- PL/42671
Batch No.- HAKT 78811
Mfg. Date- Jan. 2018
Exp. Date- Dec. 2019
M.R.P.- Rs. 49.00
(Inclusive of all taxes)
Mfd. By: COX PHARMA
SADIQ ROAD,
PATIALA
PB-147002</td>
</tr>
</table>

2. AIM- To prepare ammoniated camphor liniment I.P. (20ml)

Ingredients	Qty. prescribed	Qty. (20 ml)
Camphor	125.0 g	2.5 g
Eucalyptus oil	5.0 ml	0.1 ml
Ammonia Solution Strong	250.0 ml	5 ml
Alcohol (90%) q.s.	1000 ml	20 ml qs

Procedure: Dissolve 2.5 g of camphor and 0.1 ml of eucalyptus oil in 12 ml of alcohol (90%) and to this add 5 ml of strong ammonia solution gradually with frequent shaking. Finally, add sufficient alcohol to produce the required volume.

Uses: Rubefacient, counter irritant

Precautions:

Do not apply on broken skin.

Prevent contact with eyes.

For external use only

Storage: Keep in cool and dry place away from sunlight.

Specimen Label: The specimen label for Ammoniated Camphor Liniment I.P. (20 ml) is given as:

Ammoniated Camphor Liniment I.P. 20 ml		
Composition: **Each 5 ml contains:** Camphor - 625 mg Eucalyptus oil, Strong Ammonia Solution, Alcohol (90%) **Directions:** Apply to affected areas and massage gently 2 or 3 times a day until the condition is relieved.	**KAPLIN®** (For relief of aches, pain and sprains) KEEP THE CONTAINER TIGHTLY CLOSED FOR EXTERNAL USE ONLY KEEP OUT OF THE REACH OF CHILDREN	Mfg. Lic. No.- PL/42671 Batch No.- HAKT 78811 Mfg. Date- Jan. 2018 Exp. Date- Dec. 2019 M.R.P.- Rs. 49.00 (Inclusive of all taxes) Mfd. By: COX PHARMA SADIQ ROAD, PATIALA PB-147002

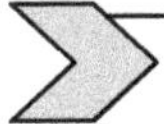 ## Linctus

Linctuses *(Synonym-Linct.)* are viscous, monophasic liquid, oral preparations usually containing high concentration of sucrose administered (for the relief of dry cough or sore throat) in small discreet dose volumes.

These syrupy or sticky preparations are intended to be sipped and swallowed slowly without dilution (i.e. without the aid of water) and contains medicaments exerting local action on the mucous membrane of the throat e.g. Codeine Linctus, paediatric B.P.C.; Codeine Linctus, Diamorphine Linctus; Compound Tolu Linctus, Paediatric; Terpin Hydrate Linctus.

Crucial Components of Linctuses

Active ingredients: Generally, sedatives and expectorants.

Vehicle: Syrup I.P./ U.S.P. (67%w/w or 85% w/v) - It exhibits sweet taste, preservative property and imparts viscosity.

Glycerin/Glycerol – It acts as demulcent (i.e. soothens the inflammed mucous membrane or skin by preventing contact with air/irritants in the surroundings), sweet in taste.

Sorbitol – It acts as sugar substitute (for diabetics) and provides viscosity to the preparation.

Invert Sugar – exhibit sweet and viscous properties.

Additives: Some additives are added to improve the stability, efficacy and palatability listed hereunder as:

Chemical stabilizers – Invert sugar has reducing action. This reduces the oxidative degradation of various colors and flavors. Hence color and flavors of fruit juices are better preserved in invert syrup.

Coloring agents: Coal tar dyes e.g. Amaranth (gives red appearance); Compound Tartrazine Solution (provides yellow appearance)

Flavoring agents: e.g. Tolu Syrup; Fruit flavors like lemon and blackcurrant; Oxymel – has acidic, honey-like sweet taste; Benzaldehyde Spirit – has almond-like flavor.

Preservatives: Syrup (67%w/w) has high osmotic pressure hence acts as self-preservative. Examples-Chloroform Spirit; Benzoic acid solution; Tolu syrup (exhibit antibacterial action due to presenece of benzoic acid and cinnamic acid)

Dosage: One or two 5 ml spoonfuls to be given 3 or 4 times a day.

Precautions: Store at a temperature not exceeding 25°C.

Formulation contains sucrose content of 85.3% and the product may be unsuitable for the diabetic patient.

Labelling Directions: To be sipped and swallowed slowly without adding water.

Protect it from direct sunlight.

Shake it well before use

Shelf-Life and Storage: These preparations have a shelf life of 36 months and should be stored in well closed air tight containers at cool place (<25°C). Store the formulations in amber colour containers if contains volatile substances.

Commercial Dispensing packs: 200 ml plastic bottle with a plastic screw cap with an aluminium foil liner/expanded polyethylene liner or 500 ml plastic bottle with a wadless plastic screw cap.

OTC/Patient packs: 100 ml or 200 ml amber glass bottle with a plastic "Jaycap" closure.

Uses: Acts as demulcent, sedative and expectorant

Commercial Examples

S.No.	Linctus (Brand Name)	Composition/Active Ingredients	Manufacturer/Company	Therapeutic Indication
1.	Codylex®	Codeine Phosphate, Chlorpheniramine	Anglo-French Drugs & Industries Ltd., India	For dry cough
2.	Comtus®	Codeine Phosphate, Chlorpheniramine Maleate, Menthol	Comed Chemicals Ltd.	For wet cough
3.	Mits® Linctus DX	Dextromethorphan	AstraZeneca Pharma India Ltd.	For wet cough; expectorant
4.	Tixylix®	Pholcodine Citrate	AHPL, India	Cough suppressant, Antitussive, Mild Sedative

Practicals Based on Linctus

1. AIM-To prepare Terpin and Codeine Linctus BP

Ingredients	Qty. prescribed (1000 ml)	Qty. used (40 ml)
Terpin hydrate BPC 1968	6.25 g	250 mg
Menthol	2 g	80 mg
Codeine Phosphate	3.2 g	128 mg
Glycerin	400 ml	16 ml
Syrup (Sucrose 1g/5 ml)	260 ml	10.4 ml
Ethanol	300 ml	12 ml
Purified water q.s.	1000 ml	40 ml

Theory: Terpin is an insect repellent. However, the cis-form hydrate is used orally expectorant and helps to loosen mucus and to ease congestion in patients presenting with acute or chronic bronchitis, and to related pulmonary conditions. It is derived from sources such as oil of turpentine, oregano, thyme and eucalyptus. Terpin hydrate (cis-p-menthane 1, 8 diol hydrate) is prepared by the action of nitric acid on oil of turpentine in the presence of alcohol. It enhances bronchial secretion directly and acts as an expectorant in productive cough by loosening the mucus. Oral ingestion of terpin hydrate linctus with empty stomach may cause nausea, vomiting, or abdominal pain. It efflorescences in dry air and exhibit solubility in water (1g in 200 ml).

Method of Preparation:

Dissolve the terpin hydrate in the alcohol; add the rest of the ingredients and sufficient quantity of purified water to make 1000 ml. Mix and filter, if necessary.

Dosage: For adults: Take 1 × 5ml spoonful, after food. Repeat after 6 hours if required, but not more than 3 doses in 24 hours.

Precautions: Do not give to children under 18 years old. Don't exceed the stated dose.

Uses: Used as expectorant, for symptomatic relief of chronic bronchitis.

Directions for use: To be taken orally only. Shake the bottle.

Storage: Do not store above 25°C. Protect from light. Keep out of the sight and reach of children.

*(**Note:** Should be contained in amber glass bottle with white 28 mm child resistant tamper evident cap with expanded polyethylene liner/Saranex liner)*

Specimen label:

Terpin and Codeine Linctus BPC 1968 40 ml		
Composition: **Each 5 ml contains:** Terpin hydrate-31.25 mg Codeine Phosphate-16 mg Menthol-10 mg in a vehicle q.s. **Dosage:** For adults: Take 1 × 5ml spoonful, after food. Repeat after 6 hours if required, but not more than 3 doses in 24 hours. **Directions:** To be taken orally only. Shake the bottle.	**TERCODIL®** Used as expectorant, for symptomatic relief of chronic bronchitis KEEP THE CONTAINER TIGHTLY CLOSED FOR EXTERNAL USE ONLY KEEP OUT OF THE REACH OF CHILDREN	Mfg. Lic. No.- PL/42671 Batch No.- HAKT 78811 Mfg. Date- Jan. 2018 Exp. Date- Dec. 2019 M.R.P.- Rs. 49.00 (Inclusive of all taxes) Mfd. By: COX PHARMA SADIQ ROAD, PATIALA PB-147002

2. AIM- To prepare Mandle's Paint B.P. 1988 (25 ml) (Synonym: Crystal Violet Paint Compound; Mandl's Paint; Pigmentum Iodine Compositum; Pig. Ind. Gp.)

Ingredients	Qty prescribed (1000 ml)	Qty. used (25 ml)
Iodine	12.5 g	312.5 mg
Potassium iodide	25.0 g	625 mg
Alcohol 90%	40.0 ml	1 ml
Water	25.0 ml	0.62 ml
Peppermint Oil	4.0 ml	0.1 ml
Glycerin q.s.	1000 ml	25 ml

Theory: Throat paints are highly viscous liquid preparations meant for application to submucosa of throat. They contain high content of glycerin which being viscous in nature, stick to the affected site for longer time and provide long lasting effect. Alcohol in the preparation being volatile in nature evaporates on exposure to air, and helps in deep penetration of medicament. Iodine and potassium iodide interact to form polyiodides which have antiseptic effects. Peppermint oil in the preparation acts as a flavoring agent.

Method of Preparation: Put the water into a 50 ml conical measure. Dissolve the potassium iodide (KI) and add the iodine and stir until completely dissolved. In a 10 ml conical measure, dissolve 0.2 ml of peppermint oil in 2 ml of alcohol (90%v/v). Using a pipette, transfer 1.76 ml to the iodine solution and mix well. Make the volume with glycerin and mix thoroughly. By difference, transfer 25 ml for dispensing.

Labelling Directions:

"Throat Paint"

"Store in a cool place" (As iodine is volatile)

"Shake the bottle" (As some of the oil separates on storage)

"Not to be swallowed in large amounts" (Alternatively this advice can be given verbally to the patient, with an explanation).

Uses: Used for treating pharyngitis and follicular tonsillitis.

(Notes: Because of the high viscosity of the vehicle, excess should be prepared since it is impossible to transfer the entire content to a bottle. In this instance, 40 ml should be made to avoid approximation, the excess is rather large but the remainder is usually kept for future use.

A glass can or a counter-balanced watch glass and a vulcanite spatula must be used for weighing the iodine and they should be washed immediately afterwards.

Care must be taken to avoid spillage during weighing preparation of the solution. This is because the bench surface can be badly stained by the dye, iodine)

<table>
<tr><td colspan="3" align="center">Mandl's Paint B.P.C. '88' (25 ml)</td></tr>
<tr>
<td valign="top">
Composition:

Each 5 ml contains:
Iodine-62.5 mg
Potassium iodide-125 mg
Alcohol (90%)
P. water- 0.124 ml
Glycerin q.s.-5 ml
Directions:
Use as directed on the label (i.e. apply 2-3 times a day) or as advised by the physician.
</td>
<td valign="top" align="center">
COX MANDL'S PAINT
Helps in the treatment of tonsils and sore throat
Helps in treating laryngitis and pharyngitis
Prevents pain caused by canker sores

Store in a cool and dry place away from direct sunlight
Shake the bottle well before use
KEEP OUT OF THE REACH OF CHILDREN
</td>
<td valign="top" align="center">
Mfg. Lic. No.- PL/42671
Batch No.- HAKT 78811
Mfg. Date- Jan. 2018
Exp. Date- Dec. 2019
M.R.P.- Rs. 49.00
(Inclusive of all taxes)

Mfd. By: COX PHARMA SADIQ ROAD, PATIALA PB-147002
</td>
</tr>
</table>

3. AIM-To prepare Codeine Linctus, Paediatric BP 1988

Ingredients	Qty. prescribed (1000 ml)	Qty. used (40 ml)
Codeine Phosphate	3g	120mg
Lemon Syrup	200ml	8ml
Benzoic acid solution	20ml	0.8ml
Chloroform Spirit	20ml	0.8ml
Purified Water	20ml	0.8ml
Compound Tartrazine Solution	10ml	0.4ml
Syrup, up to	1000ml	40ml

Method of preparation:

Codeine phosphate is weighed and taken in a conical flask. Water is added to the flask, heated gently to dissolve. Color, benzoic acid solution and chloroform spirit are added one at a time and mixed thoroughly after each addition. Lemon syrup is added and mixed. Syrup is added and mixed.

Dosage: One dessert spoonful *t.i.d*

Uses: For relieving the symptoms of cough and bronchitis.

Storage: Codeine phosphate degrades in light, so an amber color bottle is used.

Labeling Directions: "To be sipped and swallowed slowly without adding water"

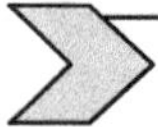

Solutions

A solution is a clear homogenous mixture that is prepared by dissolving a solid, liquid or gas in a liquid. In pharmaceutical terms, solutions are liquid preparations that contain one or more chemical substances dissolved in a suitable solvent or mixture of mutually miscible solvents.

Classification

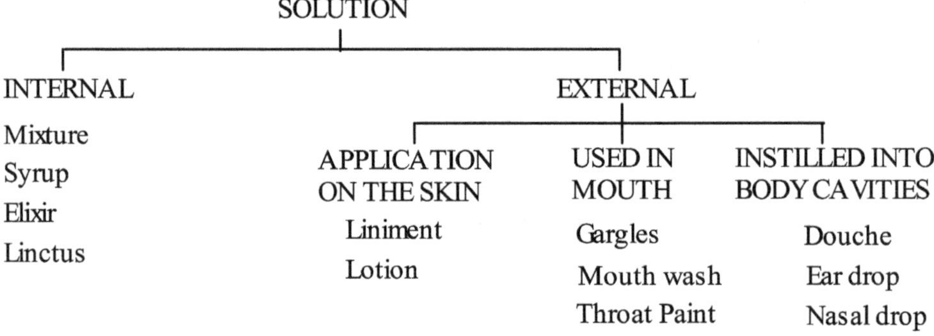

CLASSIFICATION OF SOLUTION

(i) According to the route of administration

a) *Oral solutions*—through oral route.

b) *Otic solutions*—instilled in the ears.

c) *Ophthalmic solution*—instilled in the eyes.

d) *Topical solutions*—applied over the skin surface.

(ii) According to composition and uses

a) *Syrup*—aqueous solution containing sugar.

b) *Elixir*—sweetened hydroalcoholic (combination of water and ethanol) solution.

c) *Spirit*—Solution of aromatic materials in alcohol.

d) *Aromatic Water*—Solution of aromatic material in water.

e) *Tincture / Fluid extract*—Solution prepared by extracting active constituents from crude drugs. e.g. Compound cardamom tincture. They may made up of chemical substances dissolved in alcohol or in hydroalcoholic solvent. e.g. Tincture of Iodine.

f) *Injection*—Certain solution prepared to be sterile and pyrogen-free and intended for parenteral administration.

FORMULATION CONSIDERATION

<table>
<tr><td>

1) Solubility
   a) pH
   b) Cosolvency
   c) Solubilization
   d) Complexation
   e) Hydrotrophy
   f) Chemical modification of the drug molecule

2) Preservation
   a) Preservatives
   b) Antioxidants
   c) Reducing agents
   d) Synergists

</td><td>

3) Organoleptic consideration
   a) Sweetening agents
   b) Flavoring agents
   c) Coloring agents
   d) Viscosity control
   e) Overall appearance

4) Stability
   a) Chemical stability
   b) Physical stability

</td></tr>
</table>

Practicals Based on Solutions

1. AIM- To prepare cresol with soap solution I.P. (40ml)

Ingredients	Qty prescribed (1000ml)	Qty. used (40ml)
Cresol	500ml	20ml
Vegetable oil	170g	6.8g
Oleic Acid	10ml	0.4ml
Potassium hydroxide	42g	1.68gm
Purified water q.s.	1000ml	40ml

Theory: Cresols are organic compounds which are methyl phenols. They have melting point close to room temperature and thus generally exist as liquids. They are slowly oxidized on exposure to air hence stored in air tight containers. Cresol is generally used with soap solution in which soap is incorporated to (a) impart detergent property, (b) improve natural miscibility of cresol and water by reducing critical temperature of cresol-water system, (c) sustain germicidal action of cresol and improve stability of cresol.

The free fatty acids present in vegetable oil react with (the process is called saponification) potassium hydroxide to form potassium salt of fatty acid. This salt acts as emulsifier for cresol.

Procedure:

- Dissolve potassium hydroxide in 1-2ml of purified water, and heat on water bath.

- Take vegetable oil and oleic acid, and heat on water bath at a temperature of 60°C. Separately heat cresol too.

- Now add the potassium hydroxide to oil solution with continuous stirring in small portions.
- Add cresol to the said mixture and keep on stirring until a homogenous mixture is obtained.
- Heat the solution with continuous stirring until both the solution dissolves completely and a creamy mass is formed.

Uses: Disinfectant

Precautions: For External Use Only

2. AIM- To prepare Lugol's solution or Aqueous Iodine Solution I.P.(40ml.)

Ingredients	Qty prescribed (1000ml)	Qty used (40ml)
Iodine	50.0g	2gm
Potassium iodide	100.0g	4gm
Purified water q.s.	1000.0ml	40ml

Theory- Aqueous iodine solution also known as "Lugol's solution" is an aqueous dispersion of iodine in potassium iodide solution. Iodine is insoluble in water. Therefore, it is made soluble in water by adding potassium iodide which results in formation of triiodides and poly iodides that have very high solubility in water. The preparation is used orally for supplementing iodine in the treatment of thyrotoxicosis.

Preparation: Dissolve weighed amount of potassium iodide in water. Add iodine to above solution, stir, add sufficient water to make volume upto 40ml.

Storage: Store in cool place.

Uses: Used as a source of iodine in treatment of thyrotoxicosis and goiter.

3. AIM- To prepare weak iodine solution I.P. (40ml.)

Ingredients	Qty prescribed (1000ml)	Qty used (40ml)
Iodine	50.0g	2g
Potassium iodide	100.0g	4g
Alcohol (50% v/v)	200.0ml	8g
Purified water q.s.	1000ml	40ml

Theory- Weak iodine solution also known as "tincture of iodine" is used externally as an antiseptic. It is an aqueous dispersion of iodine and potassium iodide containing small quantity of alcohol. Alcohol acts as a solubilizer as well as antiseptic.

Procedure: Dissolve iodine and potassium Iodide in sufficient amount of alcohol. Then add the alcoholic solution to sufficient water to make the volume up to 40ml.

Precautions- For external use only

Uses: Antiseptic

4. AIM- To prepare lead sub-acetate solution I.P. (40ml)

Ingredients	Qty prescribed (1000ml)	Qty used (40ml)
Lead acetate	250g	10g
Lead monoxide	175g	7g
Distilled water q.s.	1000ml	40ml

Theory: Lead sub-acetate solution is a solution made by reaction of lead acetate with lead monoxide, which is colorless, sweetish, astringent and of alkaline reaction. On exposure to air, it absorbs carbon dioxide from air forming lead carbonate which is deposited at the bottom as white precipitate. To prevent the following reaction, only distilled water is used for preparing this solution.

$$Pb_{-2} + CO_3^{2-} \rightarrow PbCO_3 \text{ (White ppt.)}$$

Procedure: Dissolve lead acetate in 30ml of distilled water. Add lead monoxide, set aside for 24h, shaking occasionally and pass through filter paper. Add sufficient water to produce required volume.

Precaution: For external use only

Uses: Mild topical Antiseptic, protective, mild astringent

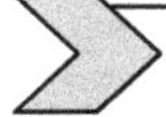 **Spirits**

They are alcoholic or hydroalcoholic solutions of volatile substances. The active ingredients may be solid, liquid or gas.

Uses: Internal, Inhalation, Flavouring agents.

Method of preparation:

1. Distillation method

2. Simple solution method

3. Solution with meceration

Practicals Based on Spirits

1. AIM- To prepare Chloroform Spirit I.P. (10 ml)

Ingredients	Qty prescribed (1000ml)	Qty. used (10ml)
Chloroform	50ml	0.5ml
Alcohol 90% q.s.	1000ml	10.0ml

Theory: Spirits are alcoholic or hydroalcoholic solutions of volatile substances. Most of them are used as flavoring agents but a few have medicinal value. The active ingredient in spirit may be solid or liquid. Spirits have to be cautiously used as flavoring vehicles because the ingredient soluble in spirits may get precipitated out when they are added to aqueous solutions due to insolubility of alcohol soluble fractions in water. Spirits are also sensitive to ions because the alcohol soluble fraction gets precipitated out in presence of ions.

Procedure: Mix about 0.5 ml of chloroform in sufficient alcohol to make up the total volume up to 10ml.

Uses: Preservative vehicle for liquid preparations.

Storage: Store at cool and dry place in an air tight container.

2. AIM- To prepare peppermint spirit B.P.C. (10ml)

Ingredients	Qty prescribed (1000ml)	Qty. used (10ml)
Peppermint Oil	100ml	1ml
Alcohol 90% q.s.	1000ml	10ml

Theory- Peppermint spirit (B.P.C) is a pharmaceutical preparation containing peppermint oil dissolved in suitable amount of alcohol. As oil is not completely soluble in alcohol so a small amount of distributing agent like talc is used which adsorbs excess of oil and provides clarity and uniformity to the formulation.

Procedure: Dissolve 1ml of peppermint oil in sufficient amount of alcohol to make the volume 10ml. Then to this solution add about 5% i.e. 0.5g of talc (sterilized talc) and allow it to stand for few hours. Then filter off the solution until clear solution is obtained.

Uses: Flavoring agent for liquid preparations

3. AIM- To prepare aromatic spirit of Ammonia USP (20ml)

Ingredients	Qty prescribed (1000ml)	Qty. used (20ml)
Ammonium Carbonate	34 g	680mg
Ammonia solution strong	36 ml	720mg
Lemon oil	10 ml	0.2ml
Lavender Oil	1 ml	0.02ml
Nutmeg oil	1 ml	0.02ml
Alcohol 90%	750 ml	15ml
Purified Water q.s.	1000 ml	20ml

Procedure: Dissolve ammonium carbonate in strong ammonia solution and 195 ml of water, and allow it to stand for 12 hours. Dissolve oils in alcohol contained in a measuring cylinder. Slowly add ammonium carbonate solution and enough water to make up 1000 ml.

Use: A respiratory stimulant.

Precaution: To be taken under medical supervision only. NOT FOR ORAL CONSUMPTION

4. AIM- To prepare spirit of ether I.P. (10ml)

Ingredients	Qty prescribed (1000ml)	Qty used (10ml)
Anesthetic ether	330ml	3.3ml
Alcohol 90% q.s.	1000ml	10ml

Procedure: Dissolve 3.3ml of ether in alcohol. Add sufficient alcohol to make up the volume up to 10 ml.

Uses: Anesthetic

Precautions- Prevent contact with eyes. NOT TO BE TAKEN ORALLY

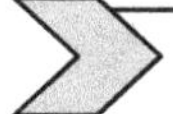 **Eye Drops**

Eye drops are sterile aqueous or oily solutions or suspensions for instillation in the eye. They are applied into the *cul-de-sac* (i.e. the space between the eye ball and eye lid).

Essential characteristics

✓ They should be sterile.
✓ They should be iso-osmotic with lachrymal secretions; i.e. the eye drops are iso-osmotic with 0.9%w/v sodium chloride solution.
✓ They should have almost neutral pH (pH 7.4).
✓ They should be free from foreign particles, fibres and filaments.
✓ They should be preserved with a suitable bactericide.
✓ They should remain stable during its storage.

Ingredients

(i) Vehicle: Purified water

(ii) Antimicrobial agents or preservatives:

(a) Phenylmercuric acetate (PMA)	–	0.002%w/v
(b) Phenylmercuric nitrate (PMN)	–	0.002%w/v
(c) Benzalkonium chloride (BAC)	–	0.01%w/v
(d) Chlorhexidine acetate	–	0.01%w/v
(e) Chlorbutol	–	0.5%w/v
(f) Thiomersal	-	0.1%w/v

(iii) Active ingredients:

Water soluble drugs: Chloramphenicol, Ciprofloxacin, Gentamicin, Pilocarpine, Atropine

Water insoluble drugs: Hydrocortisone acetate

(iv) Viscosity building agents

They are used in some special eye-drops for prolonged action of the drug; e.g.Hydroxy propyl methyl cellulose (HPMC or Hypermellose), Polyvinyl alcohol (PVA)

Procedure

Preparation of eye-drops consists of 4 – stages:

(i)   Preparation of bactericidal and fungicidal vehicles.

(ii)   Solution of the medicament(s) *(i.e. active ingredients) and if appropriate the adjuncts.

(iii) Clarification

(iv)   Sterilization

Step-I: *Preparation of vehicle*

The preservative of choice is dissolved in purified water in the prescribed concentration.

Step-II: *Solution of medicament(s) and adjuvants*

All the medicaments and adjuvants are dissolved in the antimicrobial solutions to form a stable mixture.

Step-III: *Clarification*

To remove any particulate matter, the solution is clarified by passing through membrane filter having pore size of 0.8µm. The clarified solution is immediately transferred into final containers and sealed.

Step-IV: *Sterilization*

The eye-drops are sterilized by any one of the following sterilization methods:

(a) Autoclaving done after packing the product with container.

(b) Heated at 98 to 100^0C for 30 minutes after packing the product with the container.

(c) Filtration through membrane filter (pore size 0.22µm); done after packing the product, in a sterile room and the filtered product is directly packed in containers.

Containers:

Eye drops are dispersed in neutral glass container. Either glass dropper or plastic cap-nozzle is used.

Labeling:

Eye drops should be labeled for external use only along with storage conditions to maintain full activity.

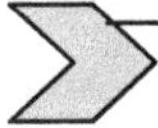

Ear Drops

Ear drops are simple solutions in which usually water is used as vehicle and in some cases, glycerol may be used due to its softening effect on wax.

They are mainly used for treating mild infections, softening wax, cleansing after infections, antisepsis, drying weeping surfaces.

Practical Based on Ear Drops

1. AIM-To prepare Phenol Glycerin ear drops

Ingredients	Quantity prescribed
Phenol Glycerin	4 ml
Glycerin q.s.	10 ml

Theory: Phenol glycerin is too strong; hence it should be diluted with glycerin before using as an antiseptic. Since water cannot be used due to the formation of phenoxide ion, glycerin serves the purpose of the base as well as a vehicle.

Procedure: Weigh 4g of phenol glycerin and add glycerin to it in a dry container upto 10 ml until both of them mix thoroughly.

Direction: Two drops to be instilled into affected ear as directed by physician.

Storage: Store in a dry place

Precautions: FOR EAR USE ONLY, NOT TO BE TAKEN ORALLY, DO NOT DILUTE WITH WATER, KEEP AWAY FROM CHIILDREN

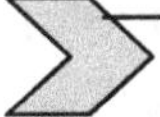

Gargles and Mouthwashes

Gargles are the aqueous solutions that are used for treating the pharynx and nasopharynx by forcing air from the lungs through the gargle which is held in the throat.

Mouthwashes are aqueous solution which is most often used for its deodorant, refreshing or antiseptic effect or for control of plaque. It may contain alcohol, glycerin, synthetic sweeteners, flavoring & coloring agents, local antiseptics etc.

Practicals Based on Gargles and Mouthwashes

1. AIM-To prepare Phenol Glycerin gargle (50 ml)

Ingredients	Qty prescribed (1000ml)	Qty used (50ml)
Phenol Glycerin	50 ml	2.5ml
Amaranth Solution (1% w/v in Chloroform Water)	10 ml	0.5ml
Purified Water q.s.	1000 ml	50ml

Theory: The low amount of phenol present in this formulation is sufficient to act as bactericide. Glycerin provides viscosity and sweetness to the preparation. This helps the preparation to remain in contact with the mucous membrane of the throat for longer time. The sweet taste and cooling sensation allow the preparation to be used as a gargle. Amaranth solution is first dissolved in chloroform water as it readily dissolves in it and it imparts a distinctive colour to the gargle.

Procedure: Prepare 1%w/v amaranth solution in chloroform water. In a separate container measure 5 ml of phenol glycerin and add 1 ml of amaranth solution to it with continuous stirring. Add sufficient amount of water to make up to 50 ml and mix thoroughly.

Direction: Dilute with equal volume of warm water before use as directed.

Storage: Store in a cool place.

Precautions: FOR EXTERNAL USE ONLY, NOT TO BE SWALLOWED.

Precautions: Prevent contact with eyes.

- Not to be swallowed in large quantities.

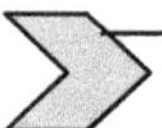

Enemas

Enemas are aqueous/oily solutions, suspensions or o/w emulsions of medicaments intended for rectal administration for cleansing, therapeutic or diagnostic purposes (to exert anthelmintic, anti-inflammatory, nutritive, purgative or sedative effects or for X-ray/ diagnostic examination of the lower bowel). The volume of the enema depends on the types of enema administered, age and condition of the patient.

Types of Enemas: Broadly enemas can be classified into three types: -

1. *Evacuant or Cleansing enemas:* Such types of enemas are used to evacuate faeces in constipation or before the surgery of the gut. These mechanisms of these enemas are mentioned hereunder:

    (i) *Stimulating peristatis:* Large volumes (~2L) are used to stimulate the peristaltic movement of colon. These enemas are warmed to body temperature (by keeping the container in warm water before use) before administration in order to avoid cold shock and discomfort to the patient. e.g. Plain enema, turpentine enema, soft soap enema

(ii) *Osmotic retention:* Such type of enemas do not exceeds 100-200 ml in volumes (used as such without warming to the body temperature) which acts by causing osmotic retention of water in the bowel. Therefore, these are also termed as *retention enemas.* e.g. Paraldehyde enema, magnesium sulphate enema, sodium chloride enema, sorbital enema, sodium phosphate enema.

(iii) *Lubricating the faecal matter:* Such types of enemas are used in volumes of 100-200 ml to lubricate the faecal matter impacted due to constipation and thus provides smooth passage in bowel. Therefore, these are also termed as *lubricating enemas* e.g. castor oil enema, olive oil enema, arachis oil enema, glycerin enema.

2. ***Therapeutic enemas:*** Such types of enemas are employed to exert local action (i.e. in conditions such as piles, inflammatory bowel disease) or systemic therapeutic effect in the lower bowel of children, bed ridden or comatose patients. Therefore, these are also termed as *medicated enemas.* E.g. sedative action (chloral hydrate, paraldehyde), antithelmentic (quassia for threadworms), anti-inflammatory (corticosteroids-ulcerative colitis, inflammatory bowel disease), nutrition (vitamins, minerals).

3. ***Diagnostic enemas:*** Such type of enemas use radioisotope labeled suspensions or solutions which are used to examine the lower bowel (in case of colonoscopy, x-ray examination) etc. e.g. barium enema using $BaSO_4$ suspension.

Directions for use: Warm up to the body temperature (37°C) before use only for large volume enemas.

Storage: Should be stored in a cool and dark place.

Containers: Stored in colored fluted glass bottle with rectal nozzle (Supplied for single use). Lubrication of nozzle is done by sodium alginate jelly or sodium carboxymethyl cellulose jelly.

Practicals Based on Enemas

1. AIM- To prepare soft soap enema (40 gm)

Ingredients	Qty. prescribed (1000 g)	Qty. used(40 g)
Soft soap*	400 g	16g
Purified water q.s.	1000 g	40g

Theory- Enemas are liquid preparations which are meant for insertion into the rectum. They are basically of three types, i.e. evacuant, therapeutic and diagnostic enemas. Soft soap is soluble in water. Soft soap enema is a large volume enema which falls under the category of retention enemas and is required to be administered in large volumes (~500ml) to exert stimulating effect on colon for relieving constipation. Such enemas need to be warmed to body temperature before administration because if it is not so, then the patient may suffer from severe hypothermia due to difference in temperature.

Method of Preparation (Simple solution method):

Dissolve 16 g of soft soap in sufficient quantity of water to make the volume equal to 40ml.

Uses: For treating severe constipation.

Storage: Store in amber colored, narrow mouthed, fluted glass bottle fitted with plastic screw cap.

Precautions-

- For rectal use only

- Warmed to 37°C before administration

- Not for oral consumption

Specimen Label:

Soft Soap Enema 40 g		
Composition: **Each 5 g contains:** Soft soap-2g Purified water- 5g Action- Lubricates and softens stool **Directions for use:** Gently insert flexible nozzle into rectum and press plunger to express contents. In resistant cases, treatment may be repeated in one hour.	**SOFEMA®** As an aid in the relief of constipation KEEP THE CONTAINER TIGHTLY CLOSED FOR EXTERNAL USE ONLY KEEP OUT OF THE REACH OF CHILDREN	Mfg. Lic. No.- PL/42671 Batch No.- HAKT 78811 Mfg. Date- Jan. 2018 Exp. Date- Dec. 2019 M.R.P.- Rs. 49.00 (Inclusive of all taxes) Mfd. By: COX PHARMA SADIQ ROAD, PATIALA PB-147002

*(*Note: The method of preparation of soft soap has been discussed in Aim No. 3 as mentioned below).*

2. AIM- To prepare paraldehyde enema (50ml).

Ingredients	Qty. Prescribed (100 ml)	Qty. (50 ml)
Paraaldehyde solution	10 ml	5 ml
Benzyl alcohol	1 ml	0.5 ml
Sodium chloride solution (0.9% w/v) qs.	100 ml	50 ml

Theory: Paraldehyde, a trimer of aldehyde (soluble in cold water) is a colourless, transparent liquid which exhibit characteristic odor. It possesses sedative, hypnotic and anticonvulsant properties. For rectal administration, freshy prepared 10% enema (isosmotic with body fluid) in physiological saline (0.9% w/v) is used.

3. AIM- To prepare soft soap USP. (50g)

Ingredients	Qty prescribed (1000g)	Qty used (50g)
Vegetable oil	380g	19g
Oleic acid	20.0g	1g
Potassium hydroxide	91.7g	4.58g
Glycerin	50.0ml	2.5g
Purified water q.s.	1000.0g	50g

Theory: Soaps are sodium or potassium salts of higher fatty acids mainly oleic acid and stearic acid. Sodium salts of fatty acids are generally known as hard soaps due to high alkalinity content whereas potassium salts of fatty acids are known as soft soaps because their alkalinity content is low. Potassium soaps can be early used on skin because the variation or difference between pH of skin i.e. 4.5 and soap have less pH which does not disrupt or cause any damage where as sodium soaps are harsh to use.

Procedure:

- Mix vegetable oil and oleic acid and heat on water bath at 60°C.
- Mix potassium hydroxide and in minimum quantity of water and heat on water bath at 60°C.
- Now slowly add potassium hydroxide solution to mixture of oils stirring continuously.
- Then add glycerin to previously heated solution to 60°C with constant stirring to produce required volume.

Uses: Laxative

Precautions- Prevent Contact With Eyes, For External Use Only

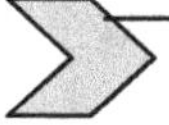

Glycerites

Glycerines (Glycerites) are solutions or mixtures of medicinal substances not less than 50% by weight of glycerine. Most of the glycerites are extremely viscous and some are jelly like.

Glycerine is used as a solvent to prepare permanent and concentrated solutions of many drugs. Some of these solutions may be used as such or may be used for diluting the alcoholic solutions of drugs which are not easily soluble in alcohol or water.

Practicals Based on Glycerites

1. AIM- To prepare Boric Acid Glycerin I.P. (30 g)

Ingredients	Quantity prescribed (1000g)	Quantity used (30g)
Boric Acid	310g	9.3g
Glycerin q.s.	1000g	30g

$$H_3BO_3 + 2\,CHOH \longrightarrow \text{(Glyceroboric acid)}$$

Theory: Boric acid reacts with glycerin to form a coordinate compound called as glyceroboric acid. Glyceroboric acid is highly viscous in nature and releases boron at a very slow rate resulting in long lasting antiseptic effect of the formulation.

Procedure: Weigh about 15g of glycerin and heat on water bath at temperature not exceeding 100°C and add about 9.3g boric acid slowly with continuous stirring. Stir vigorously until boric acid dissolves completely and a homogeneous solution is formed.

Storage: Store in an air tight container

Uses: Topical antiseptic

Precaution: For external use only

2. AIM- To prepare Tannic Acid Glycerin I.P. (30g)

Ingredients	Qty prescribed (1000g)	Qty. used (30g)
Tannic Acid	200 g	6.00 g
Sod. Citrate	10 g	0.30 g
Dried Sodium Sulfite	2 g	0.06 g
Glycerin	788 g	23.64 g

Procedure: Take tannic acid, dried sodium sulfite and sodium citrate in a porcelain dish with about ½ of glycerin mix then until smooth mixture is produced. Then add remainder of glycerin and mix well, heat the mix on water bath to temperature between 115-120°C with occasional stirring until solution is complete.

Uses: Gum paint in gum infection

Precautions: NOT TO BE SWALLOWED

3. AIM- To prepare Phenol Glycerin I.P. (30 g)

Ingredients	Quantity prescribed (1000g)	Quantity used (30g)
Phenol	160g	4.8g
Glycerin	840g	25.2g

Theory: Glycerites are liquid preparations containing minimum 50% w/w of glycerin. They contain soluble or insoluble substances and are intended for internal or external use. They are also known as "Ornamental Solution". Glycerin is used as a solvent which has following properties: -

1. Sweet in nature- suitable for oral use.

2. Highly concentrated solution can be made

3. Highly viscous in nature- long lasting effect and is thus preferred over other solvents like propylene glycol.

$$\text{C}_6\text{H}_5\text{OH} + H_2O \rightleftharpoons \text{C}_6\text{H}_5\text{O}^- + H_3O^+$$

(Phenoxide ion)

Highly Corrosive

Phenol tends to give phenoxide ion when brought in contact with water which is highly corrosive hence it is never diluted with water and stored in air tight container to prevent exposure to moisture.

Procedure: Weigh 4.8g of phenol and dissolve in 25.2g of glycerin and warm gently on water bath till both the ingredients dissolve completely.

Note- Temperature of water bath should not exceed 100°C as glycerin undergoes dehydration and forms a corrosive product acrolyene.

Storage: Keep in cool and dry place. Store in air tight container.

Uses: Antiseptic, used to treat sores. As paint for mouth ulcers and tonsillitis.

Precautions: DO NOT SWALLOW

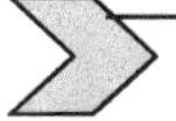

Miscellanous Systems

AIM- To prepare benzyl benzoate application I.P. (40ml)

Ingredients	Qty prescribed
Benzyl benzoate	250g
Emulsifying Wax	20g
Purified water	1000g

Theory: Benzyl benzoate application consists of benzyl benzoate as active ingredient which is an ester of benzyl alcohol and benzoic acid, prescribed for lice and scabies infestations. The active ingredient is inflammable and also should not be used on open skin. Moreover, the emulsifying wax present, as the name suggests it is an emulsifier. It consists of 1 parts of sodium lauryl sulphate with 4 parts of cetostearyl alcohol.

Procedure:

- Melt emulsifying wax, add Benzyl benzoate and mix.
- Pour the mixture into sufficient purified water to produce 40ml and stir vigorously.
- Dispense the formulation.

Uses: For treatment of Pediculosis, Scabies

Precautions-

- Do not Apply on Broken Skin
- For external use only.
- Prevent contact with eyes.
- Wash your hands thoroughly after using this medication.

Questions for viva-voice

Q1. How linctus differs from syrup in terms of formulation?

Q2. Which ingredients are added to enhance the viscosity of linctus?

Q3. Why syrups and linctus should not be stored in refrigerator?

Q4. Why liniments produce 'cooling' sensation followed by 'hot' sensation when applied to skin?

Q5. What are the various roles played by alcohol in liniment formulation?

Q6. Why liniments should not be applied to broken skin?

Q7. What is the role of ammonia solution in ammoniated camphor liniments?

Q8. What are the limitations of using elixirs as vehicles for liquid dosage forms?

Q9. What are the possible incompatibilities of elixirs?

Q10. Are preservatives necessary for elixirs?

Q11. What will be the effect on the syrup prepared above a) when it is packed in a wet bottle and stored? b) When stored either in a warm or a cold place?

Q12. Suggest the best storage conditions for syrup IP/BP.

Q13. Name the different types of syrups used in pharmacy.

Q14. State the different methods of preparing syrups.

Q15. Explain why ferrous (iron) and the phosphoric acid was heated separately?

Q16. What is cochineal and how is the colouring agent sufficiently extracted according to the BP procedure?

Q17. What is the difference between co-solvency and solubilisation? Comment on their application.

Q18. Which types of formulations can be sterilized by i). autoclaving, ii). Filteration.

Q19. Can viscous eye drops be sterilized by filteration? Why?

Q20. Name the types of drugs that can be formulated as retention enema.

Q21. Why evacuant enemas are warmed to body temperature while retention enemas are not warmed before administration?

Q22. What is the purpose of potassium hydroxide while preparing cresol with soap solution I.P.

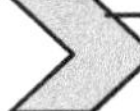

Biphasic Systems

SUSPENSIONS

A pharmaceutical suspension is a preparation where at least one of the active ingredients is suspended throughout the vehicle. In contrast to solutions, in a suspension at least one of the ingredients is not dissolved in the vehicle and so the preparation will require shaking before a dose is administered.
(Note: Blood is natural suspension)

Types of suspensions:

Diffusible suspensions: These are suspensions containing light powders which are insoluble, or only very slightly soluble in the vehicle, but which on shaking disperse evenly throughout the vehicle for long enough to allow an accurate dose to be poured.

Indiffusible suspensions: These are suspensions containing heavy powders which are insoluble in the vehicle and which on shaking do not disperse evenly throughout the vehicle long enough to allow an accurate dose to be poured. In the preparation of indiffusible suspensions, the main difference when compared to diffusible suspensions is that the vehicle must be thickened to slow down the rate at which the powder settles. This is achieved by the addition of a suspending agent.

Classification: Various literature studies have classified suspensions among diverse categories as listed below:

I. On the basis of route of administration:

1. Oral suspensions- e.g. antibiotics, paracetamol suspension, antacids

2. Topical suspensions- e.g. Calamine lotion

3. Parenteral suspensions- e.g. Procaine penicillin G, Insulin zinc suspension

II. On the basis of proportion of solid particles:

1. Dilute suspension (i.e. 2-10% w/v of solid)- e.g. cortisone acetate, prednisolone acetate

2. Concentrated suspension (containing 50% w/v of solid)- e.g. zinc oxide suspension

III. On the basis of particle size:

1. Colloidal suspensions (0.1-0.2 microns)
2. Coarse suspensions (>0.2 microns)
3. Molecular dispersion- (<1.0 nm)
4. Nanosuspension (~ 10 ng)

IV. On the basis of electro-kinetic nature of solid particles:

1. Flocculated suspension
2. Deflocculated suspension

Advantages of suspensions as dosage forms

✓ Insoluble drugs may be more palatable.

✓ Insoluble drugs may be more stable.

✓ Suspended insoluble powders are easy to swallow.

✓ The suspension format enables easy administration of bulk insoluble powders.

✓ Absorption will be quicker than solid dosage forms.

✓ High dose can be administered with high patient acceptability.

✓ Specially suited for children (pediatric) and elderly (geriatric) patients who cannot easily swallow solids.

Disadvantages of suspensions as dosage forms

✓ Preparation requires shaking before use.

✓ Accuracy of dose is likely to be less than with equivalent solution.

✓ Storage conditions can affect disperse system.

✓ Suspensions are bulky, difficult to transport and prone to container breakages.

Additives Used in Suspension Dosage Forms

1. *Wetting agents*: Some substances (e.g. sulfur, hydrocortisone etc.) are insoluble in water and are poorly wetted by it. During preparation it is difficult to disperse the clumps and the foam produced on shaking. So wetting agents are used to reduce the interfacial tension between the solid particle and the vehicle and increase wetting of the particle. e.g. alcohol, glycerin, propylene glycols, dioctyl sodium sulfosuccinate etc.

2. *Flocculating agents*: On standing for a long period the suspension may become difficult to redisperse on shaking. Therefore, controlled flocculation is required to prevent compact sediment, which is difficult to redisperse. Controlled flocculation can be produced either by, (i) electrolytes (e.g. potassium citrate, phosphate salts), (ii) surfactants, and (iii) polymers.

3. *Suspending agents/Thickening agents*: Suspending agents are the substances, which are added to a suspension to increase the viscosity of the continuous phase so that the particles remain suspended for a sufficiently long time and it becomes easy to measure an accurate dose. Due to increase in viscosity of the vehicle, the particles sediment at a much slower rate.

   e.g. methylcellulose, hydroxy propyl methyl cellulose, sodium carboxymethylcellulose etc. for internally used suspensions and bentonite, veegum etc. for externally used suspensions.

4. *Preservative*: The aqueous vehicle may be liable for bacterial growth, so a preservative should be used. e.g. benzoic acid, sodium benzoate, methylparaben, propyl paraben etc. may be used.

5. *Organoleptic additives*: Colors, sweeteners and flavoring agents may be used to make the oral suspensions more palatable.

   Colors: e.g. Amaranth, Tartrazine, Caramel, and other approved colors

   Sweeteners: e.g. Sucrose

   Flavors: e.g. Peppermint oil, Chocolate flavor, Raspberry syrup etc.

Advantages

Suspensions offer distinct advantages as follows:

1. **Stability**: Some drugs are not stable in solution form. In such cases it is necessary to prepare an insoluble form of that drug. Therefore, drugs are administered in the form of suspension. e.g. Procaine Penicillin G.

2. **Choice of solvent**: If the drug is not soluble in water and solvents other than water are not acceptable, suspension is the only choice. e.g. Parenteral corticosteroid.

3. **Mask the taste;** In some cases, drugs are made insoluble and dispensed in the form of suspension to mask the objectionable taste. e.g. Chloramphenicol base is very bitter in taste, hence the insoluble chloramphenicol palmitate is used which does not have the bitter taste

4. **Prolonged action:** Suspension has a sustaining effect, because, before absorption the solid particles should be dissolved. This takes some time. e.g. Protamine Zinc Insulin and procaine penicillin G.

5. **Bioavailability:** Drugs in suspension exhibit a higher bioavailability compared to other dosage forms (except solution) due to its large surface area, higher dissolution rate. e.g. Antacid suspensions provides immediate relief from hyperacidity than its tablet chewable tablet form.

Types of suspensions

The pharmaceutical suspension preparations are differentiated into suspensions, mixtures, magmas, gels and lotions.

Suspensions

Simple suspension is the insoluble solid dispersed in a liquid. The stability considerations suggest that the manufacture of drugs in dry form is ideal. They are reconstituted as suspensions using a suitable vehicle before administration.

Few examples are:

(i)   Dispersible tablets of antibiotic, amoxycillin (e.g. PRESSMOX)

(ii)   Procaine penicillin G powder (e.g. PENIDURE)

Gels

Gels are semisolid systems consisting of small inorganic particles suspended in a liquid medium. It consists of a network of small discrete particles. It is a two-phase system. e.g. Aluminum hydroxide gel.

Lotions

Lotions are suspensions which are intended to be applied to the unbroken skin without friction. e.g. Calamine lotion, hydrocortisone lotion.

Magmas and Milks

Magmas and milk are aqueous suspensions of insoluble, inorganic drugs and differ from gels mainly because the suspended particles are larger. when prepared they are thick and viscous and because of this, there is no need to add a suspending agent. e.g. Bentonite magma, milk of magnesia.

Mixtures

Mixtures are oral liquids containing one or more active ingredients, dissolved, suspended or dispersed in a suitable vehicle. Suspended solids may separate slowly on standing, but are easily redispersed on shaking. e.g. Kaolin mixture with pectin.

Classification of Suspensions

Based on the proportion of solids, suspensions are empirically classified as dilute or concentrated systems.

(i)   **Dilute suspensions**: Solid content 2-10% e.g. Cortisone acetate and prednisolone acetate suspension.

(ii)   **Concentrated suspensions**: Solid content 10-50% e.g. Zinc oxide suspension for external use, Procaine penicillin G injection, Antacid suspension etc.

Depending on the nature and behavior of solids suspensions are classified as flocculated and deflocculated.

Deflocculated suspension

In this system, solids are present as individual particles.

Flocculated suspension

In this system, particles aggregate themselves by physical bridging. These flocs are light, fluffy conglomerate which are held together by weak Van der Waal's forces of attraction.

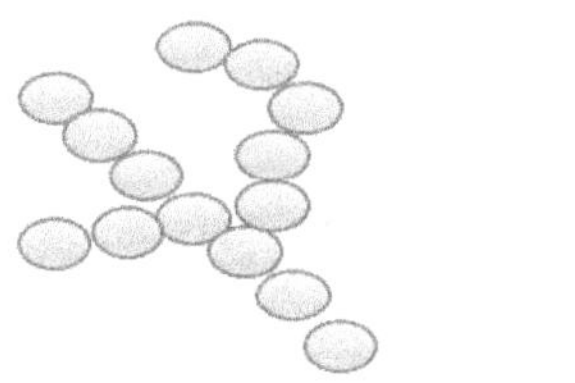
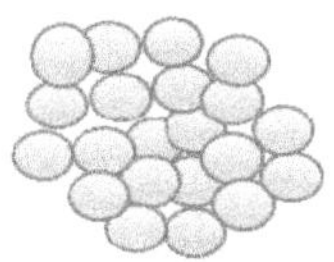

Floccule   Coagule

If the aggregate is an open network, it is called **floccule**. They are fibrous, fluffy, open network of particles. It is loosely packed after sedimentation.

If the aggregate is a closed one - it is called **coagule**. They are tightly packed, produced by surface film bonding.

Comparison between Deflocculated and Flocculated System

Deflocculated System	Flocculated System
(i) Pleasant appearance, because of uniform dispersion of particles.	(i) Somewhat unsightly sediment.
(ii) Supernatant remains cloudy.	(ii) Supernatant is clear
(iii) Particles exist as separate entities	(iii) Particles form loose aggregates.
(iv) Rate of sedimentation is slow, as the size of particles are small.	(iv) Rate is high, as flocs are the collection of smaller particles having a larger size.
(v) Particles settle independently and separately, depending on their particle size. The large particles settle first while the smaller ones settle slowly. Hence, sedimentation occurs over a long period of time.	(v) Particles settle as flocs, with small particles entagled into large particles together in flocs.
(vi) The sedimentation is closely packed and form a hard cake.	(vi) Sediment is a loosely packed network and hard cake cannot form.
(vii) The hard cake cannot be redispersed.	(vii) The sediment is easy to redisperse.
(viii)Bioavailability is higher due to large specific surface area.	(viii) Bioavailability is comparatively less due to small specific surface area.

Factors affecting the stability of a suspension

Settling in suspensions

Brownian movement

Brownian movement of particles prevents sedimentation. In general, particles are not in a state of Brownian motion in pharmaceutical suspensions, due to

(i)   larger particle size (Brownian movement is seen in particles having diameter of about 2 to 5 μm (depending on the density of the particles, the viscosity and the density of the suspending medium).

(ii)   higher viscosity of the medium.

Rate of Sedimentation-Stoke's Law

The rate of sedimentation of particles can be expressed by the Stoke's law, using the following formula:

$$\text{Sedimentation rate} = \frac{d^2 (\rho_s - \rho_l)g}{18\eta}$$

Where   d   is the particle diameter

ρ_s, ρ_l are densities of a particle and liquid respectively.

g   is the acceleration of gravity.

η is the viscosity of the medium.

Stock's law is applicable if:

(i)   particles are spherical; but particles in the suspension are largely irregular.

(ii)   Particles settle freely and independently.

In suspensions containing 0.5 - 2 % (w/v) solid, the particles do not interfere with each other during sedimentation - hence free settling occurs.

Most pharmaceutical suspensions contain 5 - 10 % or higher percentages of solid. in this cases particles interfere with one another as they fall - hence hindered settling occurs and Stoke's law no longer applies.

Stoke's law is applicable to deflocculated systems, because particles settle independently. However, this law is useful in a qualitative manner in fixing factors which can be utilized in formulation of suspensions.

Sedimemtation volume

F = Ultimate volume of sediment/total volume of suspension

- Value lies between 1 or <1 and can be >1 due to formation of flocks.
- F=1 means no sedimentation taken place
- F=0 means complete instability

1. Particle size

Rate of sedimentation ∞ (diameter of particle)^2

So smaller the particle size more stable the suspension. The particle-particle interaction results in the formation of floccules or coagules where the sedimentation rate increases. The particles are made fine either by **dry milling** prior to suspension or **wet-milling** of the final suspension in a colloid mill or a homogenizer.

2. Viscosity of the medium

According to Stoke's law:

Rate of sedimentation ∞ 1 / (viscosity of the medium)

The viscosity of suspension should be optimum. Viscosity can be increased by adding suspending agents or thickening agents. selection of high viscosity has both advantages and disadvantages.

Advantages

(i)   Sedimentation rate is retarded, hence enhances the physical stability of the suspension.

(ii) Inhibits crystal growth, because movement of particles is diminished.

(iii) Prevents the transformation of metastable crystals to stable crystals.

Disadvantages

(i)   Redispersibility of the suspension on shaking is difficult.

(ii) Pouring out of the suspension from the container may be difficult.

(iii) Creates problems in the handling of materials during manufacture.

(iv) May retard absorption of drugs from the suspension.

3. Density

Rate of sedimentation ∞ (density of solid – density of liquid medium)

Lesser the difference between the densities of solid particles and liquid medium, slower is the rate of sedimentation. Since it is very difficult to change the absolute density of the solid particles so the density of the liquid medium can be manipulated by changing the composition of the medium. The addition of nonionic substances such as sorbitol, polyvinylpyrrolidone (PVP), glycerin, sugar, or one of the polyethylene glycols or combination of these may be helpful in the manipulation.

If the density of the particles is greater than the continuous medium the particles will settle downwards, the phenomenon is known as sedimentation. If the density of particle is lesser than that of the liquid medium then the particles will move upward - the phenomenon is known as creaming.

Formulation of suspensions

The product must

1. Flow readily from the container
2. Possesses a uniform distribution of particles in each dose.

Two approaches are commonly employed to secure the two requirements,

(i) The use of structured vehicle to maintain deflocculated particles in suspension. Structured vehicles are pseudoplastic and plastic in nature; it is frequently desirable that thixotropy be associated with these two type of flow. Structured vehicles act by entrapping the particles so that, ideally no settling occurs. In reality some degree of sedimentation will usually take place. The *shear thinning* property of these vehicle does however facilitate the redispersion when shear is applied.

(ii) The application of the principles of flocculation to produce flocs that, although, they settle rapidly are easily redispersed with a minimum agitation.

Wetting of particles

The initial dispersion of an insoluble powder in a vehicle is an important step in the manufacturing process. Powders sometimes are added to the vehicle, particularly in large scale operations, by dusting on the surface of the liquid. It is frequently difficult to disperse the powder owing to an adsorbed layer of air, minute quantity of grease and other contaminants.

Powders those are not easily wetted by water and accordingly show a large contact angle, such as sulfur, charcoal and magnesium stearate are said to be *hydrophobic*. Powders those are readily wetted by water when free of adsorbed contaminants are called *hydrophilic*. e.g. zinc oxide, talc, magnesium carbonate etc. belong to this category.

When a strong affinity exists between a liquid and a solid, the liquid easily forms a film over the surface of the solid. When this affinity is non-existent or weak, the liquid faces difficulty in displacing the air or other substances surrounding the solid.

Hydrophilic solids usually can be incorporated into suspensions without the use of a wetting agent, but hydrophobic materials are extremely difficult to disperse and frequently float on the surface of the fluid owing to poor wetting of the particles or the presence of tiny air pockets on the surface of the solid particles.

To reduce the **contact angle** between solid and liquid (i.e. increase the wettability) the following agents can be tried out:

1. **Surfactants** Solid-liquid interfacial tension is reduced by incorporating a surfactant with a HLB value between 7 to 9. These are employed to allow

the displacement of air from hydrophobic material and permit the liquid, to surround the particles and provide a proper dispersion. The surfactant is mixed with the solid particles if required by shearing. The hydrocarbon chain is preferentially adsorbed to the hydrophobic surface, with the polar part of the surfactant being directed towards the aqueous phase.

2. **Hydrophilic polymers** such as sodium carboxymethyl cellulose, hydroxypropul methyl cellulose; certain water-insoluble hydrophilic material such as bentonite, aluminum-magnesium silicates, and colloidal silica, either alone or in combination can be incorporated in desired concentration. These materials are also used as suspending agents and may produce a deflocculated system particularly if used at low concentration. However, their choice depends on the route of administration of the formulation

3. **Solvents** such as alcohol, glycerol and glycols which are water miscible will reduce the liquid / air interfacial tension. The solvent will penetrate the loose agglomerates of powder by displacing the air from the pores of the individual particles thus enabling wetting by dispersion medium.

Method of selection of a suitable wetting agent

A narrow trough several inches long and made of a hydrophobic material, such as Teflon, or coated with paraffin wax can be used for the selection of suitable wetting agent. At one end of the trough is placed the powder and the other end the solution of the wetting agent. The rate of penetration of the wetting agent solution into the powder can then be observed directly. Greater the rate of penetration of the solution into the powder better is the wetting property of the solution.

Rheologic considerations

Rheologic consideration are important in

(i) the viscosity of a suspension as it affects the settling of particles. As viscosity increases rate of sedimentation of the particles reduces.

(ii) the change in flow properties of the suspension when the container is shaken and when the product is poured out off the bottle.

(iii) the spreading quality of the lotion when applied to the affected area.

(iv) during the manufacture of the suspensions.

Importance of suspending agents

The particles in a suspensions are experiencing bombardment constantly with each other owing to the Brownian movement. During this type of inter-particular interaction, the particles may circumvent the repulsive force between them and form larger particles which will then settle rapidly. Suspending agents reduce this movement of the particles by increasing the viscosity of the medium.

According to Stoke's law, The rate of sedimentation is inversely proportional to the viscosity of medium. So, the settling of the particles, either in flocculated or deflocculated system, can be slowed down by increasing the drag force on the moving particles by increasing the viscosity of the medium.

Hydrophilic polymers such as sodium carboxymethyl cellulose, certain water-insoluble hydrophilic material such as bentonite, aluminum-magnesium silicates, and colloidal silica, either alone or in combination can be incorporated in low concentration as **wetting agent.**

Hydrophilic polymers also acts as **protective colloids** and particles coated in this manner are less prone to cake than are uncoated particles.

Cellulose polymers e.g. sodium carboxymethylcellulose, methylcellulose, hydroxypropylmethylcellulose.

Proteins e.g. gelatin.

Synthetic polymer e.g. Polyacrylic acid (Carbopol)

Clays essentially hydrated aluminum and/or magnesium silicates are also useful in suspension formulation.

Characteristics of ideal suspending agent

(i)   An ideal suspending agent should have a high viscosity at negligible shear; i.e. during shelf storage; and it should have a low viscosity at high shear rates, i.e. it should be free flowing during agitation, pouring and spreading on the skin.

(ii) Suspending agents should coat the particles which will be less prone to caking than the uncoated particles.

Pseudoplastic substances e.g. tragacanth, sodium alginate and sodium carboxymethylcellulose show these desirable qualities. It is a shear thinning system, i.e. when this type of system is shaken or agitated the viscosity diminishes.

A suspending agent that is thixotropic as well as pseudoplastic should prove to be useful since it forms gel on standing and becomes fluid when disturbed. e.g. Bentonite - Carboxymethylcellulose has both pseudoplastic and thixotropic behavior.

Suspending agent	Concentration in which generally used
Sodiumcarbxymethylcellulose	0.5 − 2.5 %
Tragacanth	1.25 %
Guargum	0.5 %
Carbopol 934	0.3 %

Controlled flocculation

Assuming that the powder is properly wetted and dispersed attention may now be given to the various means by which controlled flocculation may be produced so as to *prevent compact sediment which is difficult to redisperse.* Controlled flocculation can be described in terms of the materials used to produce flocculated suspensions, namely, (i) electrolytes, (ii) surfactants, and (iii) polymers.

(i) **Electrolytes** act as flocculating agents by reducing the electric barrier between the particles, as evidenced by a decrease in the zeta-potential and formation of a bridge between adjacent particles so as to link them together in a loosely arranged structure.

Example: When bismuth subnitrate is suspended in water it has been found (by electrophoretic studies) that they possess a large positive charge, or zeta potential. Because of the strong forces of repulsion between adjacent particles, the system remains in deflocculated (peptized) state. The addition of monobasic potassium phosphate (KH_2PO_4) to the suspension causes the positive zeta-potential to decrease owing to the adsorption of the negatively charged phosphate anion. The particles then can come closer to form aggregates.

On further addition of KH_2PO_4 the zeta potential eventually falls to zero and then increases in a negative direction. Microscopic examination of the various suspensions shows that at a certain positive zeta potential, maximum flocculation occurs and will persist until the zeta potential has become sufficiently negative for deflocculation to occur once again. The onset of flocculation coincides with the maximum sedimentation volume determined. Sedimentation volume remains reasonably constant while flocculation persists, and only when the zeta potential becomes sufficiently negative to effect deflocculation.

(ii) **Surfactants** both ionic and nonionic, have been used to bring about flocculation of suspended particles. The concentration necessary to achieve this effect would appear to be critical since these compounds may also act as wetting agents to achieve dispersion.

(iii) **Polymers** are long chain, high molecular weight compounds containing active groups spaced along their length. These agents act as flocculating agents because part of the chain is adsorbed on the particle surface, with the remaining parts projecting out into the dispersion medium. Bridging between these latter portions leads to the formation of flocs.

Hydrophilic polymers also act as protective colloids and particles coated in this manner are less prone to cake than are uncoated particles.

Flocculation in structured vehicle

Although the controlled flocculation approach is capable of fulfilling the desired physical chemical requisites of a pharmaceutical suspension, the product can look unsightly if the sedimentation volume, is not close to or equal to 1. So a suspending agent is added to retard sedimentation of the flocs. Such agents as carboxymethylcellulose (CMC), Carbopol 934, Veegum, tragacanth or bentonite have been employed, either alone or in combination.

These may lead to incompatibilities, depending on

   (i)   the initial particle charge

   (ii) the charge carried by flocculating agent and

   (iii) the charge carried by suspending agent.

Preparation of suspensions

Method of preparations can be subdivided into two broad categories:

Precipitation method

There are three methods

1. organic solvent precipitation
2. precipitation effected by changing the pH of the medium and
3. double decomposition

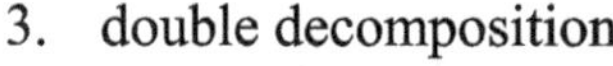

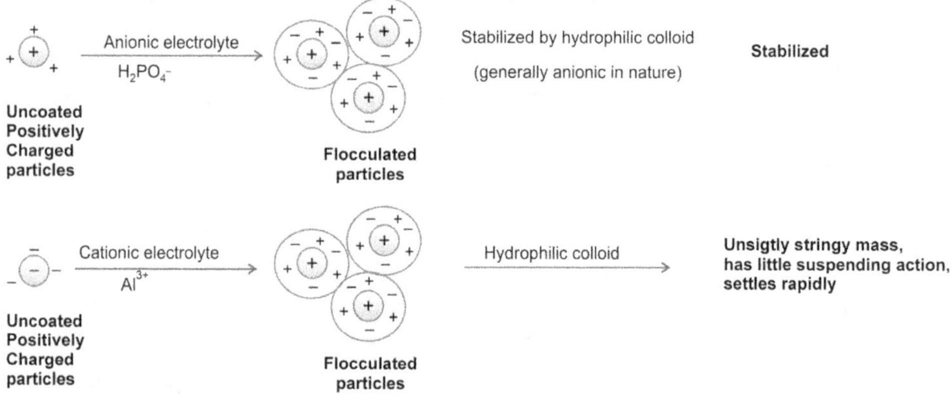

To overcome this incompatibility the following method is applied

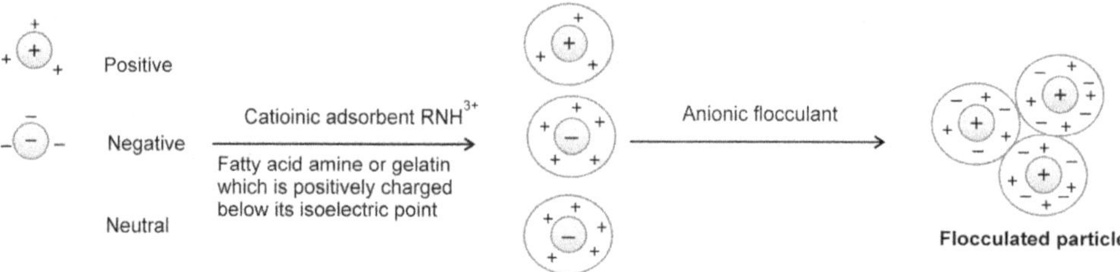

(i)   Organic solvent precipitation

Water insoluble drugs can be precipitated by dissolving them in water-miscible organic solvents (e.g. alcohol, acetone, propylene glycol and polyethylene glycol) and then adding the organic phase to distilled water under standard conditions produces a suspension having a particle size in the 1 to 5 µm range.

Example: Prednisolone is precipitated from a methanolic solution to produce a suspension in water.

Disadvantage: Harmful organic solvents may be difficult to remove.

Advantage: In case of parenteral or inhalation therapy very fine particles are required, which can be prepared by this method.

(ii) Precipitation effected by changing the pH of the medium

A drug may be readily soluble at a certain pH and precipitate at another pH. This type of drug is first dissolved in the favorable pH and then the solution is poured in another buffer system to change the pH of the medium and the drug will form a suspension in the medium of the second pH.

Example 1: Estradiol suspensions can be prepared by changing the pH of its aqueous solution; estradiol is readily soluble in alkali as potassium or sodium hydroxide solutions. If a concentrated solution of estradiol is thus prepared and added to a weakly acidic solution of hydrochloric, citric or acetic acids, under proper conditions of agitation, the estradiol is precipitated in a fine state of subdivision.

Example 2: Insulin suspension may also be prepared by pH change method. Insulin has an isoelectric point of approximately pH 5. When it is mixed with a basic protein, such as protamine, it is readily precipitated when pH is between the isoelectric points of the two components, i.e. pH 6.9 to 7.3. Protamine-Zinc-Insulin (PZI) contains an excessive quantity of zinc to retard the rate of absorption. According to the British Pharmacopoeia phosphate buffer is added to an acidified solution of PZI so that the pH is between 6.9 to 7.3 to form the suspension.

(iii) Double decomposition method

In this method two water soluble reagent forms a water insoluble product.

Example: White Lotion NF is prepared by slowly adding zinc sulfate solution in a solution of sulphurated potash to form a precipitate of zinc polysulphide.

Dispersion method

In this case the powder form of the drug is directly dispersed in the liquid medium. The liquid medium should have good power of wetting the powder.

1. Small scale preparation method

   A suspension is prepared on the small scale by grinding or levigating the insoluble material in the mortar to a smooth paste with a vehicle containing the dispersion stabilizer and gradually adding the remainder of the liquid phase in which any soluble drugs may be dissolved. The slurry is transferred to a graduated cylinder; the mortar is rinsed with successive portions of the dispersion medium is finally brought to the final volume.

2. Large scale preparation method

   On large scale dispersion method, the solid particles are suspended using ball, pebble and colloid mills. Dough mixers, pony mixers and similar apparatus are also employed.

Evaluation of Suspension Stability

Sedimentation volume

Since redispersibility is one of the major considerations in assessing the acceptability of a suspension, and since the sediment formed should be easily dispersed by moderate shaking to yield a homogeneous system, measurement of the sedimentation volume and its ease of redispersion are the two common evaluative procedures.

Definition: The sedimentation volume, F, is defined as the ratio of the final, or ultimate volume of the sediment (Vu), to the original volume of the suspension (Vo), before settling. Thus

$$F = Vu / Vo$$

The sedimentation volume can have values less than 1 to greater than 1. If the volume of sediment in a flocculated system equals the original volume of suspension, then F = 1. Such a product is said to be in 'flocculation equilibrium'.

Procedure: The suspension is taken in a measuring cylinder upto a certain height and left undisturbed. The particles will settle gradually. The value of F is determined from the ratio of the volume of the sediment at that instant of time (Vu) and the original volume of the suspension (Vo). The value of F is plotted against time (t). The plot will, will start at 1.0. at time zero. The curve will either run horizontally or gradually sloping downward to the right as time goes on.

One can compare different formulations and choose the best by observing the line, the better formulation obviously producing lines that are more horizontal and/or less steep.

If the suspension is highly concentrated then the suspension is diluted with the continuous medium (liquid phase) and then the sedimentation volume is determined.

Degree of flocculation

A more useful parameter is the degree of flocculation, β.

Definition: The degree of flocculation is the ratio of ultimate sediment volume of *flocculated* suspension to that of *a deflocculated* suspension.

$$\beta = \frac{\text{sedimentation volume of } \textit{flocculated} \text{ suspension } (F)}{\text{sedimentation volume of } \textit{deflocculated} \text{ suspension } (F\infty)}$$

$F\infty = V\infty / Vo$ $F\infty$ = sedimentation volume of *deflocculated* suspension
     $V\infty$ = ultimate sediment volume of *deflocculated*
suspension
     Vo = original volume of suspension
$F = Vu / Vo$ F = sedimentation volume of *flocculated* suspension
     Vu = ultimate sediment volume of *flocculated* suspension
Therefore, $\beta = F / F\infty$
          $= (V\infty / Vo) / (Vu / Vo)$
          $= (V\infty / Vu)$

$$\beta = \frac{\text{ultimate sediment volume of } \textit{flocculated} \text{ suspension } (Vu)}{\text{ultimate sediment volume of } \textit{deflocculated} \text{ suspension } (V\infty)}$$

Redispersibility

The evaluation of redispersibility is also important. To quantitate this parameter to some extent, a mechanical shaking device may be used. It simulates human arm motion during the shaking process and can give reproducible result when used under controlled conditions.

Rheologic methods

Rheologic behavior can also be used to help determine the settling behavior and the arrangement of the vehicle and particle structural features for purposes of comparison. The structure of the suspension changes during storage period. This structural changes can be evaluated by rheologic method.

A practical rheologic method involves the use of a Brookfield viscometer mounted on a helipath stand. The T-bar spindle is made to descend slowly into the suspension, and the dial reading on the viscometer is then a measure of the resistance the spindle meets at various level in the sediment. In this technique, the T-bar is continually changing position and measures undisturbed samples as it advances down in the suspension. This technique also indicates in which level of the suspension the structure is greater, owing to the particle agglomeration, because the T-bar descends as it rotates, and the bar is continually entering new and essentially undisturbed material.

Thus, using the T-bar spindle and the helipath, the dial reading can be plotted against the number of turns of the spindle. The result indicates how the particles are setting with time. In a screening study the better suspensions show a lesser rate of increase of dial reading with spindle turns, i.e. the curve is horizontal for a longer period.

Electrokinetic techniques

Instrument: Microelectrophoresis apparatus.

Such instrument permit measurement of the migration velocity of the particles with respect to the surface electric charge or the zeta potential. Zeta potential correlated well with the visually observed caking and certain zeta potential produced more stable suspensions because aggregation was controlled and optimized.

Particle Size Changes

During storage or transport the product may experience a fluctuation of temperature which may lead to crystal growth or physical incompatibilities. Normally it may take time to check the stability regarding crystal growth. So to accelerate this effect *freeze-thaw cycling* technique is particularly applicable. The product is put into refrigerator and again brought into room temperature — this type of temperature cycling promotes the growth of particle size. The growth of particle and size distribution are estimated by microscopic means.

Example(i) The crystal growth of sulfathiazole in suspensions is found to accelerate after temperature cycling

Example(ii) the preservative and protective colloid, may have a profound effect on the physical performance of a suspension under freeze-thaw conditions. Two low solid content steroid injectable preparations of following compositions underwent freeze-thaw condition the first preparation showed intense caking while the latter was unaffected.

Preparation	Protective colloid	Preservative	Result after freeze-thaw
I	sodium carboxy methylcellulose	benzyl alcohol	Caked badly
II	carboxy methyl cellulose	methyl paraben, propyl paraben	No caking

Example (iii) Gelatin solidifies at low temperature and methyl cellulose gets precipitates in hot water.

Practicals Based on Suspensions

1. AIM- To prepare milk of Magnesia I.P. (40ml)

Ingredients	Qty prescribed (1000ml)	Qty used (40ml)
Magnesium Sulphate	47.5g	1.9g
Sodium hydroxide	15.0g	0.6g
Light magnesium oxide	52.2g	2g
Purified water q.s.	1000.0ml	40ml

Theory: Milk and magmas are viscous aqueous suspensions of insoluble inorganic drugs. These particles are bigger than the particles of gel. When prepared they are viscous and because of this there is no need to add a suspending agent. Milk of magnesia I.P. is an antacid prepared by hydration and precipitation method where the following reaction occurs.

$$MgSO_4 + 2NaOH \longrightarrow Mg(OH)_2 + Na_2SO_4$$

$$MgO + H_2O \longrightarrow Mg(OH)_2$$

Precipitates of Magnesium hydroxide are formed which are washed to remove any sulphate ion sticking to the precipitate. The presence of sulphate ion is tested by using a solution of barium chloride, which results in formation of cloudy white precipitate of barium sulphate, if any sulphate ion is present.

$$BaCl_2 + SO_4^{2-} \longrightarrow BaSO_4 \text{ (white cloudy precipitates)} + Cl_2$$

Administration of magnesium hydroxide is also related to cause constipation, so a small amount of aluminum hydroxide is added to the preparation to decrease its effect as $Al(OH)_3$ result in loosening of stool i.e. mild laxative.

Procedure: Dissolve NaOH in 6ml of purified water, add light MgO, mix to form a smooth cream and then add sufficient water to form 125ml. Pour this suspension in a thin stream into a solution of magnesium sulphate in 125ml of purified water, stirring continuously during mixing, allow the precipitate to subside & remove the clear liquid by filtering the precipitates. Wash the precipitates with purified water until filtrate gives only a slight reaction for sulphate. Mix the washed precipitate with sufficient purified water to produce 40ml.

Uses: Antacid

2. AIM- To prepare calamine lotion I.P. (40ml)

Ingredients	Qty prescribed (1000ml)	Qty used (40ml)
Calamine	150.0g	6g
Zinc Oxide	50.0g	2g
Bentonite	30.0g	1.2g
Sodium Citrate	5.0g	0.2g
Liquefied Phenol	5.0ml	0.2ml
Glycerin	50.0ml	2ml
Rose Water q.s.	1000ml	40ml

Theory: Lotions are liquid preparations meant for external applications. Calamine lotion is a suspension of calamine which is chemically Zinc Oxide (99.5% w/w) and Ferric Oxide (0.5% w/w). Calamine lotion I.P. contains calamine as astringent, anti-infective, and antimicrobial, bentonite acts as a suspending agent, sodium citrate functions as a stabilizer, liquefied phenol is an antimicrobial, glycerin prevents drying up of skin. Calamine lotion is an antipruritic lotion which is applied on skin for various burns, rashes, minor skin infections.

Procedure: Triturate Calamine, Zinc Oxide, and Bentonite taken in ascending order by weight with a solution of sodium citrate in about 28ml of rose water. Add liquefied phenol, glycerin and sufficient rose water to make up the volume (40ml).

Uses: Topical anti-infective, Mild Astringent, treating sun burns and skin rashes.

Precautions: FOR EXTERNAL USE ONLY, SHAKE WELL BEFORE USE

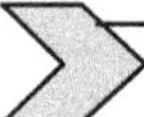 ## Emulsions

An emulsion is a thermodynamically unstable dispersed system consisting of at least two immiscible liquid phases, one of which is dispersed as globules in other liquid phases and the interface is stabilized by the presence of an *emulsifying agent*. Emulsified systems range from lotions of relatively low viscosity to ointments and creams, which are semisolid in nature. The particle diameter of the dispersed phase generally extends from about 0.1 to 10 μ and as 100 μ is not uncommon in some preparations.

Types of emulsions:

I. Ordinary emulsion systems / Primary emulsion systems / Simple emulsion systems:

- ✓ o/w type –oil dispersed in water (where oil → dispersed phase and water→ continuous phase)
- ✓ w/o type –water dispersed in oil (where water→ dispersed phase and oil→ continuous phase)

(II) Special emulsion systems:

- ✓ Multiple emulsions – (e.g. w/o/w system or o/w/o system)
- ✓ Microemulsions or Nanoemulsions

Primary Emulsions: In this system, the dispersed phase is disseminated as droplet throughout the continuous phase. Most the primary emulsions are based on o/w system and are used for oral administration. Lotions and creams may be based on o/w or w/o systems according to their use.

Multiple emulsion type

Such systems are complex and are designed in order to sustain or control the release of an active ingredient. These systems comprise of three phases: i.e. w/o/w or o/w/o (known as "emulsions within emulsions") and the active ingredient present in the innermost phase has to cross two phase-boundaries to reach the external continuous phase.

I: Continuous phase (External aqueous phase)

II: Middle oil phase

III: Inner aqueous phase

Methods of Preparation

The formulation development of emulsion involves certain quantity of energy to form the interface between the two phases, and additional work must be done to stir the system to overcome the resistance to flow. In addition, heat often is supplied to the system to melt waxy solids and /or reduce the viscosity of the oil phase. Because of the variety of oils used, emulsifying agents, phase-volume ratio and the desired physical properties of the product, a wide selection of equipment is available for preparing emulsions. Generally, at lab scale, emulsion is made using mortar (composed of glass or porcelain) and pestle using trituration process. Some of pros and cons of this approach is listed as below:

Advantages:

- ✓ Useful approach for small batches.
- ✓ Based on simple operation and low cost

Disadvantages

- ✓ Particle size obtained is relatively high.
- ✓ Applicable to only those ingredients having certain viscosity prior to trituration in order to achieve a satisfactory shear.

Other Commercial Methods

1. Agitators / Mechanical stirrers

Advantages:

✓ Useful for the emulsification of easily dispersed, low-viscosity oils.

✓ Useful for small-scale production and can be employed at lab scale.

Disadvantages:

✓ Continuous shaking tends to break up not only the phase to be dispersed but also the dispersion medium, in this way, impairs the ease of emulsification.

2. Colloid mill

Advantage

✓ Very high shearing force can be generated.

✓ Very fine particles can be prepared.

✓ Particularly useful in preparing suspensions containing poorly wetted solids.

✓ Useful for the preparation of relatively viscous emulsions.

3. Homogenizers:

The dispersion of two liquids is forced through a small orifice at high pressure. It consists of a pump that forces the dispersion at pressure of 500-5000 psi and an orifice through which this fluid impinges upon homogenization value held in place on the valve seat by a strong spring. As the pressure builds up, the spring is compressed and some of the dispersion escapes between the valve and valve seat. At the point, the energy is stored in the liquid as pressure is released and causes the product to turbulence/shear.

4. Ultrasonic devices

Advantages

✓ Useful for obtaining low viscosity and extremely low particle size.

Disadvantages

✓ Large scale production is not feasible using this technique.

COMMON TESTS FOR IDENTIFICATION OF EMULSION

S.No.	Test	Methods	Observation	Comments
1.	Dilution test	This method involves dilution of the emulsion with water. If the emulsion mixes freely with the water, it is of o/w -type. Generally, addition of disperse phase will crack an emulsion and the two phase will separate out.	Emulsion can be diluted only with external phase.	Useful for liquid emulsions only.
2.	Dye test	A small amount of a water-soluble dye (e.g. methylene blue or brilliant blue) may be dusted on the surface of the emulsion. If water is the external phase (i.e. o/w type) then the dye will be dissolved uniformly throughout the media and colorless drops will be seen. If the emulsion is of the w/o -type then particles of dye will dispersed as blue colored drops in colorless background.	Water-soluble solid dye tints only o/w emulsion. Microscopic observation usually is helpful.	May fail if ionic emulsifiers are present.

Contd....

S.No.	Test	Methods	Observation	Comments
3.	Conductivity test	This test employs a pair of electrodes connected to an external electric source and immersed in the emulsion. If the external phase is water, a current will pass through the emulsion and can be made to deflect a volt-meter needle or cause a light in the circuit to glow. If the oil is the continuous phase then the emulsion will fail to carry the current.	Electric current is conducted by o/w emulsions, owing to the presence of ionic species in water.	Fails in nonionic o/w emulsions.
4.	Fluorescence test	When an emulsion shows continuous fluorescence under a microscope after exposure to ultraviolet (UV) radiation, it is a w/o type whereas if it shows only spotty fluorescence, it is an o/w type	Since oils fluoresce under UV-light, o/w emulsions exhibit dot pattern, w/o emulsions fluoresce throughout.	Not always applicable
5.	Cobalt Chloride ($CoCl_2$) test		Filter paper impregnated with $CoCl_2$ and dried (blue) changes to pink when (o/w) emulsion is added.	May fail if emulsion is unstable or breaks in presence of electrolyte.

CRUCIAL COMPONENTS OF AN EMULSION

1. **Choice of lipid phase:** The choice of lipid phase depends on the final use of the product.

   ✓ If the oily phase itself is the active-ingredient (e.g. liquid paraffin emulsion) then the formulator has nothing to choose from.

   ✓ The active ingredient in an emulsion should not be too soluble in lipid phase, so that it affects the rate of transfer of the drug molecule to other phases.

   ✓ Externally applied (topical) emulsions should be free from any grittiness (due to variation in particle size) and should provide smoothness to the applied area. Further, emulsions normally leave a residue of the oily components on the skin after the water has evaporated. Therefore, the tactile characteristics of the combined oil phase are of great importance in determining consumer acceptance of an emulsion.

2. Phase -Volume ratio (PVR):

The ratio of the internal to the external phase is determined by the solubility of the drug and its concentration (or required dose). Apart from this criterion, PVR is normally determined by the desired consistency of the product. For a stable liquid emulsion, the limits of internal phase vary from 40 to 60%. However, the lower amounts of internal phase give a product of low viscosity with pronounced degree of *creaming* while higher percentage may produce highly viscous emulsions with tendency of *phase inversion.*

3. **Choice of emulsifying agents:** Emulsifying agents are broadly classified into three classes:

   (i)   Synthetic emulsifying agent / Surface active agents (SAA) / Surfactants (e.g. ***Anionic***-Potassium stearate, Sodium lauryl sulphate; ***Cationic***-Cetyl trimethyl ammonium bromide (or cetrimide); Ampholytic-N-dodecyl alanine; ***Non-ionic***-Sorbitan mono-oleate, (TWEEN) Polyoxyethylene sorbitan mono-oleate (Polysorbate)

   (ii) Hydrophilic colloid (e.g. ***Plant origin***-Acacia, tragacanth, alginates, chondrus and pectin; ***Animal origin***-Gelatin, egg yolk, casein, woolfat, cholesterol and lecithin; Synthetic-Methyl cellulose, Hydroxyethyl cellulose, Polyoxyethylene polymer)

   (iii) Finely divided solids (e.g. colloidal clays: bentonite (aluminium silicate) and veegum (magnesium aluminium silicate).

When an emulsifier is used alone to stabilize an emulsion − it is called *primary emulsifier.* However, in few cases, another emulsifier is used to assist the primary emulsifier in stabilizing the system − the second emulsifier is known as *auxiliary emulsifier.* Generally, emulsifiers from (ii) and (iii) category are used both as primary and auxiliary emulsifier.

The choice of emulsifier for an emulsion depends on following conditions as listed below:

✓ Should have the capacity to reduce the Surface tension $(\Upsilon) \leq 10$ dynes/cm^2 (primary emulsifiers).

✓ Ability to build a coherent film around the dispersed globules so as to prevent their coalescence (auxillary emulsifiers).

✓ Should assist in building up the zeta potential and viscosity which are essential to the stability (primary emulsifiers).

4. Consistency of Emulsion:

It plays significant role in providing stability to the emulsion. The sedimentation or creaming rate of suspended spherical particles is inversely proportional to the viscosity as per Stoke's law. For good spreadability, flowability and consistency of the emulsion, desired amount of viscosity and thixotropy is critical component of the formulation.

Alteration of viscosity in an emulsion system:

✓ Enhancing the viscosity of the continuous phase leads to increase in the viscosity of emulsion. Therefore, in o/w systems, viscosity of water is augmented by using hydrophilic colloids, gums, clays and other viscosity building agents. In w/o systems, viscosity of oil is increased by addition of polyvalent metal soaps or the use of high melting waxes and resins.

✓ Greater the PVR, the greater is the apparent viscosity.

✓ Reducing the particle size increase surface area and viscosity.

✓ Viscosity of emulsions increases upon aging. Hence, it is recommended that a newly formulated emulsion be allowed to rest undisturbed at least 24h before evaluating its viscosity.

5. **Choice of an antimicrobial preservative:**

Emulsions are prone to contamination due to presence of aqueous phase which is a good medium for microbial growth. Some ingredients, such as carbohydrates, pectin, proteins, sterols, and phosphates readily support the growth of a variety of microorganisms. As microbes may reside in both aqueous or oil phase, the preservative effective in both phases should be chosen (e.g. methyl and propyl paraben; in which methyl paraben is soluble in water while propyl and higher esters are almost water-insoluble). Some preservatives tend to interact with some ingredients. e.g. phenolic preservatives are especially susceptible to interaction with compounds containing polyoxyethylene groups. Some preservatives get solubilized, bound or complexed by the surfactants and remain inactive as preservative.

Examples: Chlorocresol, chlorobutanol, mercurials [i.e. phenyl mercuric nitrate (PMN), phenyl mercuric acetate (PMA)], esters of parahydroxy benzoate (methyl, propyl, butyl, benzyl paraben), sodium benzoateare commonly used as preservatives.

6. **Choice of antioxidants:** In an emulsion system, not only active ingredient but formulation components (e.g. unsaturated lipids) are also prone to oxidation which occurs spontaneously under mild conditions involving free radical reactions. The choice of antioxidant should be based on the kinetic measurements of fat oxidation in o/w systems in the following conditions such as:

✓ The rate of oxygen diffusion in the emulsion

✓ Pressure of oxygen

✓ Presence of trace metals if any, which act as catalysts

✓ pH of the emulsion (as oxidation is pH dependent is some cases).

Examples of agents used to prevent oxidation.

Chelating agents- Citric acid, EDTA

*Reducing agents-*Ascorbic acid, Sodium sulphite (Na_2SO_3)

Chain terminators-Water soluble compounds e.g. Cystine HCl, Thioglycollic acid

Lipid soluble compounds -e.g. Alkyl gallates (octyl, propyl, dodecyl), BHT, BHA

CAUSES OF INSTABILITY OF EMULSION

An emulsion is regarded as physically stable, if its globules retain their inherent character and remain uniformly distributed throughout the continuous phase. Under the influence of time and temperature dependent processes during storage, an emulsion's instability may be caused by- creaming, flocculation, coalescence.

1. **Creaming:** Creaming is the upward or downward movement of dispersed droplets related to the continuous phase due to the difference of density between two phases. *(Note: The downward creaming is also called sedimentation. Generally, the term "sedimentation" is associated with the downward movement of solid particles in suspension).*

   It is undesirable property for a stable emulsion, however it may be accepted if the ingredients are reconstituted by modest shaking.

   Rate of creaming can be reduced by following corrections:
   ✓ Reduction of droplet size ($<0.1\mu$, if possible)
   ✓ Reducing the difference in density between the two phases*(Note: According to Stokes Law, no creaming is possible if the specific gravities of the two phases are equal)*
   ✓ increase in the viscosity of the continuous phase

2. Flocculation

Flocculation is reversible aggregation of droplets of the internal phase in the form of three-dimensional clusters. In the floccules the droplets remain aggregated, but intact. The droplets can remain intact when the mechanical or electrical barrier is sufficient to prevent droplet coalescence.

e.g. if an insufficient amount of emulsifier is present, emulsion droplets aggregate and coalesce.

The reversibility of this type of aggregation depends on the strength of the interaction between particles, as determined by:
✓ Chemical nature of the emulsifier,
✓ Phase volume ratio
✓ Concentration of dissolved substances, especially electrolytes.

3. Coalescence

Coalescence is a growth process during which the emulsified particles join to form larger particles. Any evidence for the formation of larger droplets by merger of smaller droplets suggests that the emulsion will eventually separate completely. The major factor which prevents coalescence in flocculated and deflocculated emulsions is the mechanical strength of the interfacial barrier. Any factor or agent (e.g. *addition of a chemical, bacterial growth, temperature change*) that will destroy the interfacial film will crack the emulsion.

Other Physical Parameters

The other parameters commonly used to assess the effect of stress conditions on emulsions:

✓ Phase separation,

✓ Viscosity,

✓ Electrophoretic properties (Zeta Potential)

✓ Particle size analysis (Using Zeta Sizer) and particle count (Using Coulter count method).

Practical Based on Emulsions

1. AIM- To prepare Turpentine Liniment I.P. (40ml)

Ingredients	Qty prescribed (1000 ml)	Qty. used (40 ml)
Soft Soap	90.0g	3.6g
Camphor	50.0g	2.0g
Turpentine Oil	650.0ml	2.6ml
Purified water q.s.	1000.0ml	40.0ml

Theory: Turpentine liniment I.P. contains turpentine oil and camphor both of which are volatile in nature. The formulation involves the use of soft soap as emulsifier for forming o/w type emulsion.

Procedure:

✓ Mix soft soap with 4ml of purified water and separately make a solution of camphor in freshly rectified turpentine oil.

✓ Gradually add the camphor solution to soap mixture with trituration until thick creamy emulsion is formed. Add sufficient amount purified water to produce required volume, mix.

Therapeutic Use: Rubefacient, mild topical analgesic.

Storage: Store in a cool and dry place.

Labelling Directions: Shake the bottle well before use.
Precautions: FOR EXTERNAL USE ONLY

2. AIM-To prepare Liquid Paraffin emulsion BP (40 ml)

Ingredients	Qty. Prescribed (100 ml)	Qty. (40 ml)
Liquid Paraffin	50 ml	20 ml
Vanillin	50 mg	20 mg
Cholorform	0.25 ml	0.1
Benzoic acid	2 ml	0.8 ml
Methyl cellulose 20 (2% w/v)	2g	0.8 g
Sacchrin Sodium	5 mg	2.0 mg
Water qs.	100ml	40 ml

Theory: Methyl cellulose 20 at a concentration of 2% w/v acts an emulsing agent for the mineral oil, liquid paraffin. A primary emulsion is not required. Benzoic acid and chloroform act as preservatives and vanillin and saccharin sodium act as flavoring agent and sweeting agent respectively.

(Note: The amount of saccharin sodium is not weighable on class B dispensing balance and will be obtained by trituration using water as diluent (act as a vehicle). Trituraton of the sodium saccharin: (Sodium saccharin ~100mg is diluted with water up to 100ml; therefore, 5 ml of water will contain 5 mg of saccharin sodium).

Therapeutic Use: A lubricant laxative for chronic constipation

Procedure: Firstly, prepare a mucilage by mixing methylcellulose (20) with a about six times its weight of boiling water and allow to stand for 30 minutes to hydrate. Add an equal weight (~15 g) of ice and stir mechanically until the mucilage is homogenous. Dissolve the vanillin in the benzoic acid solution and chloroform. Add this mixture to the mucilage and stir for 5 minutes. Make the saccharin sodium titration and stir the appropriate volume of mucilage up to 50 ml.

Storage: Store in a cool and dry place. Should remain stable on storage however, a 4 week expiry/ shelf life is recommended.

Labelling Directions: Shake the bottle well before use.

Precautions: Should not be taken within 30 minutes of meal and preferably on as empty stomach. High fiber and fluid intake is recommended.

3. AIM- To prepare castor oil emulsion (Dry gum method) I.P. (10ml)

Ingredients	Qty prescribed
Castor oil	3.00ml
Tragacanth gum	0.75g
Water q.s.	10.0ml

Theory- Castor oil emulsion, a disperse system of two immiscible liquids namely castor oil and water is widely used as laxative, whereas tragacanth gum present in the prescription used as an emulsifier forming a o/w type of emulsion. Castor oil is an irritant that helps in easy defecation. And hence the formulation is used as laxative. A primary emulsion is prepared by two methods either *dry gum* or *wet gum* method.

In dry gum method, the oil is triturated with gum to hydrate it and their water is added slowly with trituration, Whereas, **in wet gum method**, the gum is first hydrated to form a mucilage and as mucilage works as an auxiliary emulsifier, oil is then added slowly, followed by final addition of water to form an o/w type of emulsion. (*Note: The ratio of oil: water: gum used for the primary emulsion will vary with the type of oil used in the formulation*)

Although, the preparation can be prepared by any of the methods, the overall therapeutic effect of the formulation is same but "DRY GUM METHOD IS CONSIDERED BETTER BECAUSE IT CAN BE EASILY MADE IN SHORT PERIOD OF TIME". On the other hand, Stability wise "WET GUM METHOD IS PREFFERED" because in this method the gum is hydrated resulting in formation of mucilage which acts as a very good emulsifying agent leading to greater stability and hence longer shelf life of the formulation.

Procedure:

✓ First primary emulsion is prepared by taking oil, water and gum in ratio of 4:2:1 respectively i.e. 12ml of oil, 6ml of water and 3g of gum.

✓ In dry gum method, gum is taken and oil is added and then 6ml of water is added drop wise with trituration.

✓ Clicking sound during trituration indicates the formation of primary emulsion.

✓ Then add remaining 34ml of water drop wise with trituration to form final emulsion.

Uses: A laxative (gastrointestinal irritant)

Labelling Instructions: Shake the bottle well before use

Storage: Store it in cool place and should not be frozen.

4. AIM- To prepare castor oil emulsion (wet gum method) I.P. (40ml)

Ingredients	Qty prescribed	Qty. used
Castor oil	3 ml	12 ml
Tragacanth gum	0.75g	3 g
Purified Water q.s.	10 ml	40 ml

Theory: Castor oil is a fixed oil that requires the addition of tragacanth gum as an emulsifying agent. The proportions are 4 oil: 2 water: 1 gum. Therefore, 12 ml of castor oil, 40 ml of water and 3 g of gum will be used to prepare the primary emulsion

Procedure:

- First primary emulsion is prepared by taking oil, water and gum in the ratio of 4:2:1 i.e. 12ml of oil, 6ml of water and 3g of gum.

- In wet gum method, gum is taken and 6ml of water is added and then 12ml of oil is added drop wise with trituration. Clicking sound comes and indicates formation of primary emulsion.

- Then add remaining 34ml of water drop wise with trituration to form final emulsion.

Therapeutic use: Act as stimulant laxative for chronic constipation

Labelling instructions: This is an unofficial formula and should be labeled as 'Castor oil 30%v/v emulsion' shake the bottle well before use.

Dosage: A normal dose is 10 ml three times a day (t.i.d) with or without food.

Storage: Store in cool a dry place, if freshly prepared shelf life of 2-3 weeks is applicable. (*Note: Should not be frozen*).

Different excipients used in liquid dosage form

S.no	Name of Excipient	Category	Trade name	Functions
1.	Acacia	Water soluble	Gum Arabic	Emulsifying agent (10–20%), Pastille base (10–30%), Suspending agent (5–10%)
2.	Adipic acid	Slightly soluble in water	Inipol DS	Acidifying agent, buffering agent, flavoring agent.
3.	Alcohol	Antimicrobial preservative	Ethanolum	Antimicrobial preservative (5-10%), Disinfectant (60–90%)
4	Ascorbyl palmitate	Water insoluble	Ascorbylis palmitas	Antioxidant (0.05%w/v)
5	Benzoic acid	Water soluble antimicrobial preservative	Acidum benzoicum	As preservative (0.1-0.2%)
6	Butylated hydroxyanisole	Water insoluble	Nipanox BHA;	Antioxidant (0.002-0.5%)
7	Butylated hydroxyl toluene	Water insoluble	Embanox BHT	Antioxidant (0.009-0.1%)
8	Calcium phosphate, tribasic	Very Slightly soluble in water	Tri-Cafos	Anticaking agent, buffering agent, dietary supplement, glidant, tablet and capsule diluent.

Contd....

S.no	Name of Excipient	Category	Trade name	Functions
9	Chlorbutanol	Water soluble antimicrobial preservative	Sedaform	In ophthalmic or parenteral dosage forms (0.5%w/v)
10	Citric acid monohydrate	Water soluble	Acidum citricum monohydricum	Acidifying agent, antioxidant, buffering agent (0.1-2.0%), chelating agent (0.3-2%), flavor enhancer (0.3-2%), preservative.
11	Ethyl acetate	Water insoluble	Ethyl ester	Flavoring agent, solvent.
12	Glycerin	Solvent, humectant, emollient	Croderol	Solvent for parenteral formulations ($\leq$50%), Humectant ($\leq$30%)
13	Hydroxyethyl cellulose	Nonionic water-soluble polymer	Cellosize HEC	Coating agent, suspending agent, thickening agent, viscosifier.
14	Isopropyl alchol	Water soluble solvent	Isopropanol	Disinfectant, solvent.
15	Maleic acid	Water soluble	Acidum maleicum	Buffering agent
16	Monobasic sodium phosphate	Water soluble	Kalipol 32	Buffering agent, emulsifying agent, sequestering agent.
17	Polysorbate 20	nonionic surfactant	Armotan PML 20	Emulsifying agent (1–15%), Solubilizing agent (1–15%), Wetting agent (0.1–3%)
18	Propyl gallate	Water insoluble	Progallin P	Antioxidant (0.002-0.1%)
19	Propyl paraben	Water soluble antimicrobial preservative	Aseptoform P	As preservative (0.05-0.2%)
20	Propylene glycol	Diluent	Propylenglycolum	Solvent (10-60%), Preservatives (15-30%), Humectant ($\approx$15%)
21	Seasame oil	Water insoluble	Lipovol SES	Oleaginous vehicle, solvent.

Contd....

S.no	Name of Excipient	Category	Trade name	Functions
22	Sodium acetate	Water soluble	sodium ethanoate.	Antimicrobial preservative, buffering agent, flavoring agent, stabilizing agent.
23	Sodium lauryl sulphate	Anionic surfactant	Elfan 240	Anionic emulsifier (0.5–2.5%), Detergent (10%), Skin cleanser in topical applications (1%), Solubilizer >0.0025%
24	Sorbic acid	Antimicrobial preservative.	Sorbistat K	In oral and topical pharmaceutical formulations (0.05–0.5% w/v)
25	Sorbitan monolaurate	nonionic surfactant	Arlacel 20	Emulsifying agent (1–15%) Solubilizing agent (1–10%) Wetting agent (0.1–3%)
26	Thimerosal	Water soluble antimicrobial preservative; antiseptic.	Thimerosal Sigmaultra	As preservative (0.001–0.15%)
27	Tocopherol	Water soluble	Aquasol E	Antioxidant, solubilizing agent
28	Tragacanth	Water insoluble	Gum tragacanth	Suspending agent, viscosifier, Emulsifying agents
29	Triethanolamine	Alkalizing agent, emulsifying agent	Tealan	As emulsifier (2–4% v/v)
30	Xanthum gum	Anionic water-soluble emulsifier	Xanthan gum	Gelling agent, stabilizing agent, suspending agent, Viscosifier

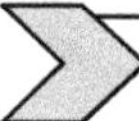

Questions for Viva-voce

Answer the following questions:

Q1.   Emulsions are thermodynamically unstable. Why?

Q2.   Differentiate between creaming and cracking.

Q3.   Distinguish between the roles of primary and auxillary emulsifiers.

Q4.   Discuss the parameters evaluated for testing the stability of emulsions.

Q5.   Enumerate the advantages of emulsions as a dosage form.

Q6.   What is phase inversion? Enumerate the cause of phase inversion.

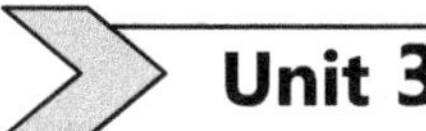 **Unit 3**

Solid Dosage Forms

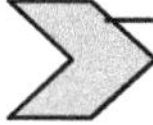 **Pharmaceutical Powders and Granules**

A powder is defined as a solid material in a finely divided particles intended for administration by mouth. They are usually mixed with water before administration. But some oral powders for veterinary use are administered by mixing with animal ration. Furthermore, most raw materials required in the preparation of tablets and capsules are available as powders, which are compressed into the tablet dosage form after granulation process.

Classification

On the basis of their size: (i.e. ability to pass through a mesh aperture):

✓ Coarse Powder

✓ Moderately Coarse Powder

✓ Moderately Fine Powder

✓ Fine Powder

✓ Very Fine Powder

✓ Ultra-Fine Powder

On the basis of therapeutic use: powders can also be classified:

✓ Bulk powder for internal use

✓ Bulk powder for external use, e.g. dusting powders and insufflations

✓ Divided powders (i.e. single dose)

Preparation of Bulk powders for internal use

Whenever several powder ingredients are present, the powders are mixed in ascending order of bulk in a mortar. At each addition, a quantity that is approximately equal the bulk already existed in the mortar is added e.g.

Compound Calcium Carbonate Powder		Compound Sodium Chloride & Dextrose Powder	
Sodium bicarbonate	37.5g	Sodium chloride	0.50g
Calcium carbonate	37.5g	Potassium chloride	0.75g
Heavy Magnesium carbonate	12.5g	Sodium carbonate	0.75g
Light Kaolin	12.5g	Dextrose	20.0g
Directions for use: Prescribed amount is dissolved in required amount of water and taken orally. *Container*: Kept in a well-closed, air tight container			

Bulk powder for external use

Classification:

A. Dusting powder   (i) Medical dusting powder (ii) Surgical dusting powder

B. Insufflations

C. Dentifrices (tooth powder)

A (i) Medical dusting powder

These are used for superficial skin conditions. They are not sterile. They are not applied on open wounds or broken skin.

Ingredients: Purified Talc, Light kaolin, Starch etc. They contain powdered drugs. Talc, kaolin are mineral ingredients. They may be contaminated with spores of *Clostridium tetani* and *Clostridium welchii*. So talc or kaolin must be sterilized by heating at 160^0C for one hour.

Preparation:

After mixing the powders in a mortar it is passed through mesh no. 120 sieve to remove gritty particles. Then it is packed in a suitable container.

Container: Dusting powder is packed inside a *sifter-top* container. (It is a container with holes in the cap. Whenever the container is shaken the powders are spread on the skin.)

Example:

Starch salicylic acid dusting powder	
Starch, in powder	75g
Zinc oxide	20g
Salicylic acid, in powder	5g

A(ii) Surgical dusting powder

These are used in body cavities and major wounds, on burns and on the umbilical cords of newborns, hence they must be sterile.

They often contain an antibacterial agent and the diluent may be sterilized i.e. maize starch.

Example: Chlorhexidine B.P.C., Hexachlorophene B.P.C.

B. Insufflations

Finely divided powders intended for application to body cavities such as tooth socket, ears, nose, vagina and throat are known as insufflations. Apparatus used to deliver a stream of finely divided powder particles to the site of application is called an *insufflator*.

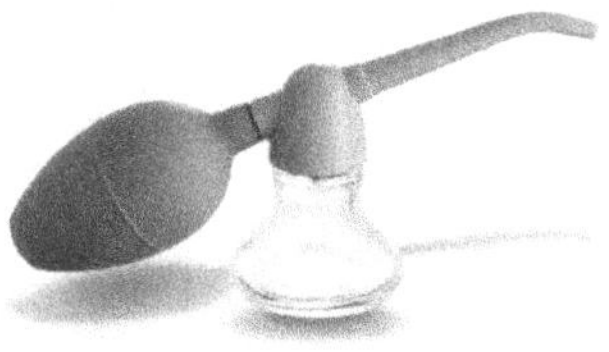

Insufflator

They are used to produce either –

(a) a local effect, as in the treatment of ear, nose and throat infections with antibiotics, or

(b) a systemic effect, from a drug that is destroyed in the intestine.

The diluent used in nasal mucosa is lactose and that used on open wound is sterilizable maize starch.

Container: Well-closed container supplied with an insufflator instrument.

The required dose of powder is taken in the container of the insufflator and with the bulb a pressure is given to force the powder through the nozzle.

Storage: With moisture the nozzle of the insufflator may get choked hence, the powder must be kept in a dry place and in a well closed container.

C. Dentifrices (tooth powders)

Powders used to clean the teeth are called *dentifrices*. It is applied with a tooth brush. They contain

(i)   a suitable detergent – hard soap powder

(ii) a suitable abrasive agent – calcium sulfate, magnesium carbonate, dibasic calcium phosphate

(iii) Sweetening agent – sodium saccharin

(iv) Flavoring agent – peppermint oil, clove oil etc.

Packaging: Sifter top metallic or plastic container.

Divided powders (i.e. single dose)

In this form of powder, each dose is separately enclosed in a piece of paper.

Classification:

(a) *Simple powder*:   Contains only one ingredient.

(b) *Compound powder*: Contains more than one ingredient.

The total amount in each dose should not be less than 120 mg so that the powder is large enough to be handled conveniently.

Packing:

1. For wrapping divided powders, white glazed paper (demy paper) is generally used.

2. The powder wrappers are stacked in a paper box and dispensed.

3. Some time *double wrapping* is required, especially if the powder is hygroscopic. In this case waxed paper is used as inner wrapper, then the demi wrapper as the outer wrapper.

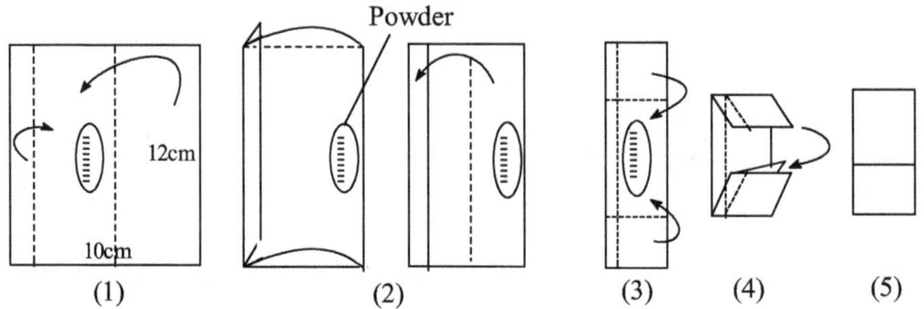

General method of preparation of powders:

1. Spatulation: If the solids form eutectic mixture, they form liquid on trituration. In this case they should be mixed lightly with a spatula.

2. Trituration: The solids are taken in a mortar and triturated with a pestle. This method reduced the particles and at the same time mixes the powders.

3. Geometric dilution: This method is used when very small amount of potent drug is to be mixed with large amount of diluent. The method can be explained with an example:

   For example, say 100mg of a potent drug (A) is to be mixed with 900mg of diluent (B), then the geometric dilution method is as follows:

   (i)   100mg A   + 100mg B   → 200mg mixture

   (ii)   200mg mixture   + 200mg B   → 400mg mixture

   (iii) 400mg mixture   + 400mg B   → 800mg mixture

   (iv)   800mg mixture   + rest of B   → 1000mg mixture

Practical Based on Powders and Granules

1. AIM- To prepare compound tragacanth powder I.P. (5g)

Ingredients	Qty prescribed (1000g)	Qty used (5g)
Tragacanth	150g	0.75g
Acacia	200g	1g
Starch	200g	1g
Sucrose	450g	2.25g

Theory: Tragacanth is a gum obtained by exudation from stem of *Astragalus gummifer*. It is employed in pharmacy as a suspending agent in mixtures containing resinous tinctures and heavy insoluble powders or to emulsify volatile oils. Mucilage of tragacanth and compound powder of tragacanth are used for these purposes, the later combining suspending power of tragacanth and gum acacia, while starch present tends to prevent agglomeration of deposit. It is also widely used as a suspending agent, emulsifier, stabilizer and also a thickener and binder.

Procedure:

- Mix all the ingredients in ascending order and triturate till fine powder is formed.

- Mixing in ascending order is required so that all the ingredients get evenly distributed in formulation resulting in formation of a uniform and homogenous product.

Uses: Pharmaceutical Aid - Emulsifier, Stabilizer, Thickener, Suspending agent.

2. AIM- To prepare Codeine Phosphate Powder (10mg)

Ingredients	Qty prescribed (100mg)	Qty used (10mg)
Codeine Phosphate	10mg	1mg
Calcium Carbonate q.s.	100mg	10mg

Theory: Calcium carbonate is used as a diluent along with codeine phosphate as it is difficult to administer such a small quantity as such. To increase the bulk of the medicament calcium carbonate is added which is inert in nature and does not react with the active ingredient.

Calculations and Procedure: For dispensing 9 doses. First calculate the amount of active ingredient for (9+1) 10 doses

   i.e.   10 mg $\times 10 = 100$ mg

Now take 900 mg of Calcium carbonate and mix calcium carbonate with Codeine phosphate according to gradual dilution

Dispense nine doses of the product in double wrapped paper.

Uses: Antitussive, Analgesic

Storage: Store at cool and dry place

Precaution: Not for children below 6 years of age.

3. AIM- To prepare hyoscine hydrobromide powder (0.6 mg) (dispense 12 doses)

Ingredients	Qty. Prescribed
Hyoscine hydrobromide	0.6mg
Lactose q.s.	100mg

Lactose is used as a diluent.

Calculations & Procedure:

- Hyoscine hydrobromide for single dose = 0.6 mg
- Calculate for (12+3) 15 doses = 0.6 mg × 15 = 9 mg. (This quantity is still not weighable)
- Triturate 100 mg of hyoscine hydrobromide with 900 mg of lactose to form 1000 mg of triturate.
- Each 100 mg of this triturate has 10 mg of Hyoscine hydrobromide, so for taking 9 mg of Hyoscine hydrobromide take 90 mg of the triturated powder.
- Mix 90 mg of triturated powder with 1410 mg of lactose to form 1500 mg of powder.
- Weigh 100 mg of the final formulation 12 times and pack in double wrapped pouches.

Uses: To treat nausea, Motion sickness.

Different excipients used in solid dosage form

S. No.	Name of Excipient	Category	Trade name	Function
1.	Alginic acid	Water insoluble	Kelacid	Release-modifying agent, stabilizing agent, suspending agent, sustained release agent, tablet binder, tablet disintegrate, taste masking agent, viscosity-increasing agent.
2	Carrageenan	Water soluble	Grindsted	Emulsifying agent, gel base, stabilizing agent, suspending agent, sustained-release agent, viscosity-increasing agent.
3	Cellulose acetate phthalate	Water insoluble	Aquacoat	Coating agent (0.5-9%)
4.	Cellulose derivatives	Water insoluble diluent	Emcocel	Adsorbent; suspending agent; tablet and capsule diluent; tablet Disintegrate.
5	Ceratonia	Water soluble	Microfleur	Controlled-release agent, stabilizing agent, suspending agent, tablet binder, viscosity-increasing agent.
6	Corn starch	Water insoluble	StarCap 1500	Binding agent, compression aid, disintegrate, tablet and capsule diluent, tablet and capsule filler.

Contd...

S. No.	Name of Excipient	Category	Trade name	Function
7	Gelatin	Water soluble	Cryogel	Coating agent, film-forming agent, gelling agent, suspending agent, tablet binder, viscosity-increasing agent.
8	Glyceryl behenate	Water soluble	Compritol 888 ATO	Coating agent, tablet binder, tablet and capsule lubricant, thickening agent, viscosity-increasing agent.
9	Hydroxypropyl starch	Partially soluble in water	Hydroxyl propyl starch	Binding agent, disintegrate, emulsifying agent, thickening agent, viscosity-increasing agent.
10.	Lactose	Water soluble diluent	Pharmatose DCL 21	Dry powder inhaler carrier, lyophilization aid, tablet binder, tablet and capsule diluent, tablet and capsule filler.
11	Maltol	Water soluble	Palatone	Flavoring agent (sweet flavor).
12	Mannitol	Water soluble diluent	Mannogem	Diluent (10-90% w/w), carrier for lyophilized preparations (20-90% w/w),
13	Menthol	Partially soluble in water	Hexahydro thymol	Flavoring agent (peppermint flavor)
14	Mysteric acid	Water insoluble	Edenor C14	Tablet and capsule lubricant.
15	Palmitic acid	Water insoluble	Emersol 140	tablet and capsule lubricant.
16	Poloxamer	Water insoluble	Lutrol	Dispersing agent, emulsifying agent, solubilizing agent, tablet lubricant, wetting agent.
17	Polycarbophil	Water insoluble	Noveon AA-1	Adsorbent, bioadhesive material, controlled-release agent, emulsifying agent, suspending agent, tablet binder, thickening agent.
18	Polydextrose	Water soluble	Litesse	Coating agent, diluent, granulation aid, humectant, tablet and capsule diluent, tablet binder, tablet filler, viscosity-increasing agent.
19	Polyvinyl Acetate Phthalate	Water insoluble coating agent	Opaseal	enteric coating agent (9-10%), Sugar coating (28-29%)

Contd…

S. No.	Name of Excipient	Category	Trade name	Function
20	Povidone	Water soluble	Kollidon	Carrier for drugs (10–25%), Dispersing agent (Up to 5%), Eye drops (2–10%), Suspending agent (Up to 5%), Tablet binder, tablet diluent, or coating agent (0.5–5%)
21	Shellac	Water insoluble	CertiSeal FC 300A	Coating agent; encapsulating agent; film-forming agent; matrix forming agent; modified-release agent.
22	Starch	Water insoluble diluent	Perfectamyl D6PH	Glidant; tablet and capsule diluent (3-25% w/w), tablet binder (3-20% w/w), Powder flow modifier (3-10% w/w)
23	Sucrose	Water soluble diluent	Saccharose	Tablet binder (50-67% w/w), Dry binder (220% w/w), coating agent (50-67% w/w)
24	Talc	Water insoluble	Altalc	Anticaking agent, glidant, tablet and capsule diluent, tablet and capsule lubricant.
25	Vanillin	Soluble in organic solvents	Rhovanil	Flavoring agent (vanilla flavor)
26	Zein	Water insoluble	Amazein	Tablet coating agent (15%), Tablet sealer (20%), Wet granulation binder (30%)
27	Zinx sterate	Water insoluble	Cecavon	Tablet and capsule lubricant.

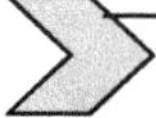

Questions for viva-voce

Answer the following questions:

Q1. Enumerate the advantages and disadvantages of powders.

Q2. Distinguish between effervescent and efflorescent powders.

Q3. Distinguish between amorphous and crystalline solids.

Q4. What are hygroscopic powders? How are they dispersed?

Q5. What is meant by double wrapping of powder?

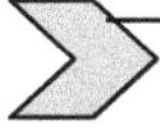 **Suppositories**

Suppositories are solid, single unit dosage forms specially designed of various shapes, weights volume and consistency adapted for rectal, urethral or vaginal (known as pessaries) administration. Suppositories may melt or dissolve (depending on the type of base used) in the rectum. These dosage forms often contain one or more active substances dispersed or dissolved in a suitable base which may be soluble or dispersible in water or melt at body temperature (or when come in contact with mucous secretions). The medicament or the base in the suppository may act as a protectant or palliative to the local tissues at the point of introduction or as a carrier of therapeutic agents for systemic or local action. Few excipients other than base and drug may be added, if necessary, such as diluents, adsorbents, surface-active agents, lubricants, antimicrobial preservatives and FDA approved coloring agents.

'Pessaries' is a kind of a suppository intended for vaginal use only having larger size moulds (4-8 g). Most of the pessaries are made exclusively for local use primarily vaginitis (inflammation of vagina caused by *E. coli*, a pathogen or due to old age i.e. dryness in vaginal mucosa due to change in pH, less secretions due to menopause) and leucorrhea (unpleasant vaginal discharge). (*Note:* In some conditions, prostaglandin pessaries are used to exert systemic effect). Some drugs used in official pessaries include- (e.g. *acetarsol*-antiprotozoal agent, *diiodohydroxyquinoline*-yeast and protoplast infections, *lactic acid-* used in leucorrhoea, *nystatin* yeast infections, *crystal violet-* anti-microbial use).

Types of Suppositories

1. Rectal suppositories
   - ✓ Approx. weight of ~2g with tapered at one or both ends (*For pediatrics-* size is less and weight ~1g).
   - ✓ Rectal insertion for local and systemic purposes.

2. Pessaries (Vaginal suppositories):
   - ✓ Approx. weight of ≥ 3-6 g or more with conical, rod-shaped or wedge shapes.
   - ✓ Exclusively used for local action on vagina

3. Urethral Suppositories (or Urethral bougies)
   - ✓ Approx. weight of ~2-4 g (size of 5-12 cm) for insertion to urethra.
   - ✓ Rarely used in practice.

4. Nasal suppositories (Nasal bougies)
   - ✓ Approx. weight of ~1 g (size of 9-10 cm) for insertion to nasal cavity.
   - ✓ Formulated only with glycerol-gelatin base and exhibit similarity with urethral bougies due to shape

5. Ear cones (aurinaria)

- ✓ Exclusively used for insertion to ear cavity
- ✓ Formulated with cocoa butter base in urethral bougies mould and cut according to the required size.

Purposes of Suppositories as a Dosage Form

- ❖ ***Lubrication Action:*** Useful as a mechanical or lubricating aid for promoting evacuation of bowel (by irritating the mucous membrane of the rectum (e.g. glycerol and bisacodyl).

- ❖ ***Local use:*** Useful for smoothening the rectal mucosa (e.g. ZnO), exert local anesthetic action (e.g. Cinchocaine, benzocaine) or astringent action (e.g. bismuth subgallate, hamamelis extract and tannic acid) or anti-inflammatory action (e.g. hydrocortisone and its acetate).

- ❖ ***Alternate route of drug delivery for certain drugs:*** The lower portion of the rectum affords a large absorption surface area from which the soluble substances can absorb and reach the systemic circulation. Drugs which irritate the GIT, causes vomiting, destroyed by the hepatic circulation, or prone to acidic or enzymatic conditions, in the stomach are well suited for alternate route of delivery for systemic action. ***Examples of drugs administered using rectal route-*** *aminophylline* (for asthmatic and chronic bronchitis), morphine (analgesic), ergotamine tartrate (for treating migraine), indomethacin and phenylbutazone (for analgesic and anti-inflammatory action).

- ❖ ***Use of Rectal route for systemic treatment is of prime significance:***

  For pediatric (such as infants) and geriatric patients (who are bed-ridden i.e. unconscious, mentally disturbed) or unable to endure oral medication because of vomiting or pathological conditions of the alimentary tract.

Disadvantages

- ✓ Low patient compliance in certain patients due to unacceptability to use
- ✓ Difficult to self-administer by arthritic or physically compromised patients.
- ✓ Unpredictable and variable absorption *in vivo.*

Factors Influencing Drug Absorption from Rectum Suppositories

Physiological factors:

The rectum is the terminal end of the intestine, begins at the rectosigmoid junction and ends at anus. Its length is 15cm. it contains a small amount of mucus which has a pH of 7.2-7.4.

The rectum has no primary absorptive functions (as villi are absent). But diffusion takes place through the rectal epithelium which is lipoidal in character. The venous flow contributes mainly to the transport of drugs. The venous flow of rectum consists of:

(i)   the inferior haemorrhoidal vein near the anal sphincter.

(ii) middle haemorrhoidal vein, which receives blood from the capillaries of the middle region of the rectum.

(iii) Superior haemorrhoidal vein which drains the upper rectal end.

The inferior and middle haemorrhoidal veins drain directly into the vena cava, thus bypassing the portal system.

The superior vein drains into the mesenteric vein which empties into the portal vein. This venous system gives rise to the assumption that drug administered in the rectum go directly to the vena cava, bypassing the liver.

The almost neutral pH of the rectal mucus (7.2) has little buffer capacity and thus the medication that is dissolved in these fluids determines the pH of the environment. If adjustment of pH is critical for efficient absorption of the medicament, suitable buffering agents may be added.

Physicochemical factors

1. *Lipid/water solubility of drug*:

   Oil soluble drugs in oily base shows slow release and slow absorption.

   Water soluble drugs in oily base shows fast release and faster absorption.

   Thus, for faster onset of action, water soluble drugs & oily base and for gradual release of drug, oil soluble form is used.

   e.g. Absorption of salicylic acid and sodium salicylate from oily base and water-soluble base.

   Salicylic acid and sodium salicylate absorption equal from oily base and salicylic acid absorption increases from water soluble base.

   e.g. Water-soluble barbiturate salt in oily base shows rapid onset of action than in water soluble base.

   e.g. Procaine HCl shows rapid onset of action when incorporated as a suspension in a fatty base.

2. *Use of surface-active agents:*

   Basically, they alter the mucus lining of the rectal ampulla with which absorption of drugs increases. The surface-active agents may also act as solubilizing agents, thus increase the absorption.

   e.g.

   (i) Ephedrine HCl, Aminophenazone, Butalbital in witepsol and cocoa butter bases containing emulsifiers above HLB 10 shows optimum release.

   (ii) Salts of phenobarbital are absorbed more readily (by rabbits) if the base contains surfactants.

(iii) Chloramphenicol incorporated in water soluble base with sodium lauryl sulfate (SLS) and polysorbates (HLB 10) showed increase in the release. Only SLS showed increase in antibiotic activity of the drug.

In case of **nonionic surfactants**, there is decreased absorption of sulfonamides due to entrapment of the drug in micelles of large sizes.

Suppository Base: A base is a vehicle made from substances (like gelatin or cocoa butter) that surrounds the drug and gets melted at body temperature and lead to slow drug release.

Class of suppository bases: As per USP, generally six classes of suppository bases have been defined:

Melting Bases:

(i) Cocoa butter

(ii) Cocoa butter substitutes

Non- Melting Bases:

(i) Glycerinated gelatin

(ii) Polyethylene glycol base

Miscellaneous Bases:

(i) Surfactant base

(ii) Tableted suppositories or inserts

1. **Melting Bases–** The bases which melt at body temperature. e.g. cocoa butter (i.e. theobroma oil).

Cocoa butter: A yellowish-white solid with a chocolate-like odour composed of glyceryl esters of stearic, palmitic, oleic and other fatty acids.

PROS:

✓ Melting range of 30 to 36 ^{0}C (i.e. solid at R.T. but melts at body temperature).

✓ Rapid liquefaction and setting on warming and cooling.

✓ Good miscibility and blandness (i.e. does not produce irritation)

CONS:

✓ Polymorphism

✓ Mould Adherence

✓ Low softening point in hot climates

✓ Melting point reduced by soluble ingredients

✓ Slow deterioration during storage

✓ Poor water absorbing capacity

✓ Leakage from the body orifices

✓ High cost

Cocoa butter substitutes (synthetic fats): These fats act as substitutes of cocoa butter which are made by hydrogenation (saturates the unsaturated fatty acid) and subsequent heat treatment (breakdown triglycerides into fatty acids and partial esters i.e. mono- and di-glycerides) of vegetable oils e.g. palm oil, arachis oil coconut oil, palm kernel oil, stearic and a mixture of oleic and stearic acids.

Advantages

✓ Solidifying points are unaffected by overheating.

✓ Resistant to oxidation

✓ Don't undergo polymorphism

✓ Good emulsifying and water absorbing capacities (due to presence of glycerides)

✓ Undergo contraction on cooling thus gets easily out of mould without lubrication

✓ Lead to transparent, odourless and elegant suppositories.

Disadvantages

✓ Become brittle on subsequent cooling (0.05 % polysorbate 80 is added to reduce brittleness)

✓ Exhibit higher fluidity and high sedimentation rate (Thickeners such as magnesium stearate, bentonite and colloidal silicon dioxide are added)

2. **Aqueous Bases**: – The bases which gets dissolve or disperse in rectal secretion, e.g. Glycero-gelatin base, and Polyethylene glycol base (PEG 400, 1000, 4000, 6000), Macrogol bases (400, 1000, 1540, 4000, 6000)

Glycero-gelatin base:

• A hydrophilic base of glycerol and water mixed to form a jelly like mass by adding gelatin.

• Slowly release of drug in the aqueous secretions (Base is well adapted for drugs like belladonna extract, boric acid, chloral hydrate, bromides, iodides, iodoform).

• Depending upon the compatibility of the drugs used, a suitable type of gelatin is selected for the purpose. Two types of gelatins are used as suppository base: Pharmagel A (made by acid hydrolysis (has isoelectric point~ 7 to 9 and act a cationic agent, being most effective at pH 7 to 8) is used for acidic drugs and Pharmgel B (made by alkaline hydrolysis (isoelectric point~ 4.7 to 5 and acts as an anionic agent, being most effective at pH 7 to 8) is used for alkaline drugs.

Limitations:

✓ Hygroscopicity and laxative properties of glycerol

✓ Incompatible with drugs those precipitate with the protein e.g. tannic acid, ferric chloride, gallic acid

✓ Difficult to handle and formulate as liquefaction time depends on the content and quality of the gelatin.

Polyethylene glycol bases/Macrogol bases (Carbowaxes): **PROS vs COCOA BUTTER**

✓ High melting point (>42^{0}C), and does not require cool storage conditions.

✓ Don't melt in the body cavities, rather slowly dissolve and disperse the drug.

✓ Non-adherence to the mould and undergo contraction on cooling.

3. **Emulsifying bases:** Some of the synthetic bases and a few proprietary bases which are commonly used include- e.g. *Witepsol* (triglycerides of saturated vegetable acids), *Massa Esterium (mixture of* di-, tri- and mono-glycerides of saturated fatty acids), *Massuppol (a* glyceryl ester of lauric acid) Fattibase® (triglycerides from palm, palm kernel, and coconut oils) Wecobee® series-FS, M, R, and S (triglycerides of coconut oil), Dehydag®, Hydrokote®, and Suppocire®.

Pros vs. Cocoa butter:

✓ No polymorphism or change in physical attributes due to over heating

✓ Rapid solidification and Non-adherence with the mould

✓ Less prone to rancidity and easily dispersible in aqueous media

Ideal properties of a suppository base:

✓ Chemically inert and physically stable for use and storage at room temperature conditions

✓ Non-reactive, odor free, elegant texture and compatibility with diverse array of drugs and auxiliary agents

✓ Nontoxic, non-sensitizing, and nonirritating to sensitive tissues

✓ Expansion–contraction characteristics such that it shrinks just enough on cooling so that it releases easily from suppository molds

✓ Melts or dissolves in the intended body orifice to release the drug

✓ Nonbinding with drugs

✓ Mixes with or absorbs some water

✓ Viscosity low enough when melted to pour easily but high enough to suspend particles of solid drug

✓ Ability to melt at body temperature or dissolve or disperse in body fluids

✓ Ease of drug release from the base without any mould adherence

✓ Retaining its shape while handling

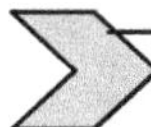

Displacement Value (DV)

The number of parts of medicament (drug) that displaces one part by weight of the base is known as the displacement value (DV) of that drug. In simpler terms, it is the amount of drug (g) that displaces 1 gram of the base. The displacement value is constant for a drug and a base.

Mathematical expression:

Displacement value (DV) of a drug

$$= \frac{\text{Amount of drug (g)}}{\text{Amount of base (g) displaced by the drug}}$$

General Method for determining DV of a drug:

The displacement value of a given drug can be determined as follows:

✓ Assume 6 suppositories prepared with theobroma oil (or any base) & their total weight $= a$ mg

✓ 6 suppositories are prepared containing 40% of the drug and their total weight $= b$ mg.

✓ Amount of theobroma oil required will be $= c$ mg $= 60\%$ of b mg $= 0.6 \times b$ mg

✓ Amount of drug required will be $= d$ mg $= 40\%$ of b mg $= 0.4 \times b$ mg

✓ The weight of theobroma oil displaced by d mg of drug $= (a - c)$ mg

✓ Displacement value of the drug $= d / (a - c)$ mg

Example:

Weight of six unmediated suppositories $= 6$g

Weight of six suppositories containing 40% of zinc oxide $= 8.8$ g

Theobroma oil in this $= \dfrac{60}{100} \times 8.8 = 5.28$ mg

Zinc oxide in this $= \dfrac{40}{100} \times 8.8 = 3.52$ mg

Theobroma oil displaced by 3.52 g of zinc oxide $= 6 - 5.28 = 0.72$ g

Therefore, the displacement value of zinc oxide $= 3.52 / 0.72 = 5$ (approx.)

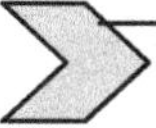

Need for Displacement Value

The volume of a suppository from a particular mould is uniform but its weight will vary because the densities of medicaments usually differ from the density of the base with which the mould was calibrated. When bases other than cocoa butter is used, or when the density factor for a drug in cocoa butter is not known, then the density factor can be estimated by calculation or experimentally determined by the double casting technique.

To prepare products accurately, allowance must be made for the change in density of the mass due to added medicaments. For this purpose, the DV of a medicament is taken into consideration. The list of DV with reference to cocoa butter, for substances prescribed in suppositories and pessaries is given here under:

Drugs/Base	DV	Drugs/Base	DV
Aminophylline	1.5	Hydrocortisone acetate	1.5
Bismuth subgallate	3.0	Ichthammol	1.0
Castor oil	1.0	Morphine Hydrochloride	1.5
Chloral hydrate	1.5	Phenobarbitone	1.0
Cinchocaine Hydrochloride	1.5	Resorcinol	1.0
Cocaine hydrochloride	1.5	Tannic acid	1.0
Hydrocortisone	1.5	Zinc oxide	5.0

Example-I: *Calculate the displacement value of Zinc oxide in cocoa butter suppositories containing 40% zinc oxide and is prepared in 1g mould. The weight of 8 zinc oxide suppository is 11.74g.*

Solution:

Weight of 1 suppository of pure cocoa butter base, $w1 = 1g$

Weight of 1 suppository of 40%ZnO suppository $= 11.74g/8 = 1.4675g$.

Amount of ZnO present in 1 suppository $= 40\%$ of $1.4675g = \dfrac{40}{100} \times 1.4675g$

$= 0.40 \times 1.4675g = 0.587g$

Amount of cocoa butter present in 1 suppository, $w2 = 60\%$ of $1.4675g =$

$\dfrac{60}{100} \times 1.4675g = 0.60 \times 1.4675g = 0.8805g$

Therefore, amount of cocoa butter displaced

$=$ Weight of 1 pure cocoa butter suppository $-$ Weight of cocoa butter present in 1 zinc oxide suppository

$= 1g - 0.8805g$

$= 0.1195g$

From definition, the displacement value of zinc oxide

$$= \dfrac{\text{Amount of drug (g)}}{\text{Amount of base (g) displaced by the drug}} = \dfrac{0.587\ \text{(g)}}{0.1195\,g} = 4.9 \approx 5\ Ans.$$

Calculation of Overage in Suppository Base Using Displacement Values:

Example I: Prepare and dispense suppositories using official (standard) formula given below and calculate the quantity of base per suppository (Hard fat BP):

Formula Ingredients	1 suppository (in mg)
Bismuth Subgallate BP	200
Resorcinol BP	60
Zinc Oxide BP	120
Castor Oil BP	60
Base	Qs

Calculations:

Step 1: Calculate the amount of each ingredient for 10 suppositories to allow for losses during preparation.

Bismuth Subgallate BP	2.0 g
Resorcinol BP	0.6 g
Zinc Oxide BP	1.2 g
Castor Oil BP	0.6 g
Base	Qs

Step 2: Use displacement values of the ingredients from literature:

Bismuth Subgallate BP	2.7
Resorcinol BP	1.5
Zinc Oxide BP	4.7
Castor Oil BP	1.0

Step 3:

Bismuth Sub-gallate BP displaces $2 \div 2.7$ g Hard Fat BP = 0.74 g

Resorcinol BP displaces $0.6 \div 1.5$ g Hard Fat BP = 0.4 g

Zinc Oxide BP displaces $1.2 \div 4.7$ g Hard Fat BP = 0.26 g

Castor Oil BP displaces $0.6 \div 1$ g Hard Fat BP = 0.6 g

The amount of base required = $(10 \times 1 \text{ g}) - (0.74 + 0.4 + 0.26 + 0.6)$

$$= 10 - 2.00$$

$$= 8.00 \text{ g}$$

Therefore, the working formula will be:

Formula Ingredients	10 suppositories
Bismuth Subgallate BP	2.0 g
Resorcinol BP	600 mg
Zinc Oxide BP	1.2 g
Castor Oil BP	600 mg
Hard fat	8 g

Example II: To prepare ten suppositories each containing 300 mg bismuth subgallate. (Given: Mould size is 1 g. Displacement value of bismuth subgallate is 3)

Solution:

300 mg bismuth subgallate = 0.3 g bismuth subgallate

Displacement value of bismuth subgallate means 3 g bismuth subgallate displaces 1 g theobroma oil.

Therefore, 0.3 g bismuth subgallate will displace

$(1 \div 3) \times 0.3 = 0.1$ g suppository base (i.e. theobroma oil)

So the working formula for each suppository will be

Bismuth subgallate	0.3g
Theobroma oil	0.9g
Total	1.2g

General Method of Preparation of Suppositories

Suppositories are prepared extemporaneously by two processes: *moulding* (hot process or fusion process i.e. drug is mixed into the molten mass, then poured at a suitable temperature into moulds and allowed to cool until set.) and *cold compression* (incorporating the medicaments into the base)

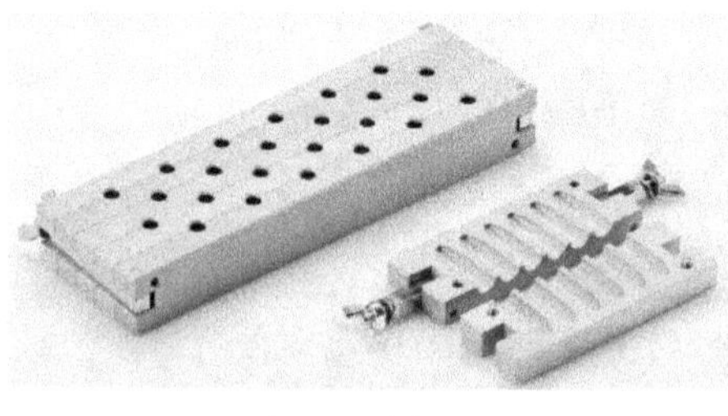

(Moulds)

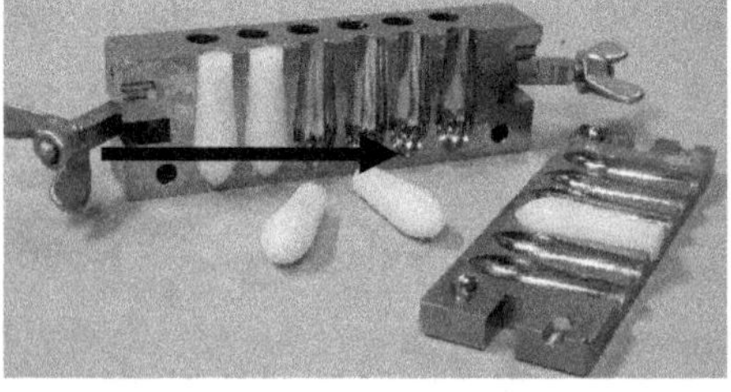

(Prepared suppositories)

Mould: Among various types and capacities (commonly 1g, 2g, 4g and 8g) of suppository moulds (made up of stainless steel, nickel-copper alloy, brass, aluminium or plastic) available, suppository moulds with *six* or *twelve* cavities with desired shape and size are generally used. For large scale production moulds up to 500 cavities may be used.

For cleaning, lubrication (*Note*-Aqueous lubricant for cocoa butter suppositories, oily lubricant for glycerol-gelatin suppositories, no lubricant is required for macrogol bases) and removal of suppositories the mould can be opened longitudinally by removing the screw in the centre of the plates.

Calibration of Mould

Suppository moulds are calibrated in terms of the weight of Theobroma Oil BP each will contain. Typical sizes are 1 g, 2 g or 4 g. Since the moulds are filled volumetrically, use of a base other than Theobroma Oil BP will require recalibration of the moulds. Many synthetic fats have been formulated to match the specific gravity of Theobroma Oil BP and therefore the mould sizing will be the same and not require recalibration. However, this is not the case for all synthetic bases. To recalibrate a suppository mould, the compounder needs to prepare a number (e.g. five) of (perfectly formed) suppositories containing only the base. These can be weighed and the total weight divided by the number of suppositories present to find the mould calibration value.

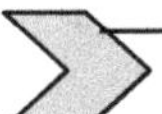 **Practical Based on Suppositories**

1. **AIM-To prepare 12 suppositories using a glycerol-gelatin base BP using a 4 g mould (calibration value 4.0)**

Ingredients	Qty. prescribed
Drug (Ichthammol)	10%
Gelatin	14%
Glycerol	70%
Water qs.	Up to 100%

Theory: These bases are mixture of glycerol and water stiffened with gelatin. The most common base used comprises of 14% w/w of gelatin and 70% w/w glycerol. In hot climates, the gelatin content could be increased to 18 % w/w. (Note: Gelatin - Pharmaceutical grade available as A and B, is a purified protein obtained from hydrolysis of collagenous tissues. It must be heat treated during the preparation to ensure that the product is pathogen free). It is more difficult to handle than other bases.

Procedure: *Preparation of glycero-gelatin suppositories*:

✓ Calculate for 14 suppositories to allow wastage. Glycero-gelatin base is 1.2 times denser than cocoa-butter base.

✓ Mould calibration for glycerol-gelatin base is 4.0 × 1.2= 4.8 g.

✓ A displacement value is not required because the drug is expressed as a percentage. However, to get the displacement value of any other drug in glycero-gelatin base

$$= \frac{\text{Displacement value of the drug in cocoa butter base}}{1.2}$$

✓ The formula for the base will be gelatin = 14 g, glycerol = 70 g and water qs. up to 100 g. The formula for the suppositories is drug = 10% w/w and glycerol-gelatin base = 90% w/w.

✓ The total weight required to prepare the suppositories is 14 × 4.8 = 67.2 g. For ease of calculation prepare 70 g. Therefore, the quantities for drug and base to be taken will be 7 g and 63 g respectively.

✓ The moulds are cleaned and lubricated with either liquid paraffin or arachis oil. The mould is kept in inverted position.

✓ Glycerol is heated to 100^0C on a water bath.

✓ In another beaker water soluble ingredients (thermostable) are dissolved and heated on another water bath. Gelatin is added to water to wet the material. Gelatin is added to water with gentle stirring. Heated on a boiling water bath until all the gelatin goes into solution.

✓ The beaker is weighed and water is either evaporated or more water is added to make up the volume.

✓ The molten mass is poured into the moulds and chilled in a refrigerator.

Storage: Each suppository is packed in thin aluminium foil and placed inside partitioned, rigid paper boxes. Hygroscopic suppositories such as glycero-gelatin suppositories should be placed in airtight jars.

Labelling directions:

'Store in a cool place only',   'For Rectal Use Only'

Precautions: May cause rectal irritation due to physiological effect of base (contains small amount of liquid).

2. AIM- To prepare Cocoa butter suppository

Preparation of cocoa butter suppositories:

1. *Lubrication of moulds*: The moulds cleaned are lubricated by aqueous lubricant (Soft soap + glycerol + alcohol). After lubrication the moulds are kept inverted to drain out excess lubricant.

2. *Melting of the base*: The cocoa butter is weighed and grated with a spatula and taken in a beaker and heated on a water bath. When about 2/3 portion of cocoa butter oil was melted, the beaker was taken out of the water bath and the solid residue was mixed and melted with a spatula. [N.B. Over heating may occur if the base is left over the heat until completely melted.]

3. About half of the melted base is added to the powdered drug on the ointment tile and levigated with the spatula to mix it smoothly. When the base is solidified, it is softened by holding the tile over the water bath for few seconds.

4. The dispersion is transferred in the beaker again and stirred gently to form a homogeneous mixture. Stirring is continued until the mixture begins to thicken. The cavities of the mould are filled up with the dispersion. The mould is left for two to three minutes until the mass just set, in then the mould is scrapped with a sharp knife. The mould is left in a cool place for 10 to 15 minutes. Then the mould is opened and suppositories are removed.

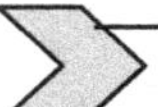 **Questions for Viva-voce**

Answer the following questions:

Q1. What is polymorphism? How does it affect cocoa butter while being formulated into suppositories?

Q2. Define displacement value and mention its importance.

Q3. Why cocoa butter is not used for pessaries?

Q4. How can the premature melting of cocoa butter suppositories be prevented?

Q5. Which types of drugs can be formulated in pessaries?

Q6. How first-pass hepatic metabolism is avoided by delivering drug in suppositories?

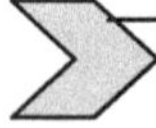 # Unit 4

Pharmaceutical Incompatibilities

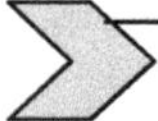 ## Definition

When two or more ingredients of a prescription are mixed together, the undesired change that may take place in the physical, chemical or therapeutic properties of the medicament is termed as *incompatibility*.

Classification

Incompatibilities are of three types:
1. Physical incompatibility
2. Chemical incompatibility
3. Therapeutic incompatibility

Physico-Chemical Incompatibilities

Physical incompatibilities:

Where the incompatibility is caused by immiscibility, solubility or liquefaction or solubilization.

Chemical incompatibilities: Where incompatibility is due to a chemical reaction or complexation.

Physical Incompatibility

It may cause unsightly, non-uniform products from which removal of an accurate dose is very difficult.

Immiscibility

1. *Problem*: Oils are immiscible with water.

   Remedy: Emulsification or solubilization.

   e.g. *Preparation of castor oil emulsion.*

   Castor oil is not soluble in water. Hence, a third agent (gum acacia) is added to prepare a stable emulsion. This third agent is called emulsifier.

   e.g. *Preparation of cresol soap solution*

CLASSIFICATION OF INCOMPATIBILITIES

PHYSICAL

- ❖ Insolubility
  - Addition of KI to solubilize I_2 in water
- ❖ Immiscibility
  - O/W or W/O type emulsions
- ❖ Liquefaction
  - Formation of Eutectic Mixture of camphor and Menthol
- ❖ Physical Degradation
  - Conversion of β form of Theobroma oil to α form.
- ❖ Physical Complexation
  - Between PEG 400 and Phenol
- ❖ Effervescence
  - Mg. Carbonate and Citric Acid
- ❖ Precipitation
  - Alkaline substances and alkaloids

CHEMICAL

- ❖ Oxidation Reduction
  - Sodium Salicylate and Sodium Bicarbonate
- ❖ Hydrolysis
  - Peniciline G sodium hydrolysis in acidic media
- ❖ Photolysis
  - Darkening of Morphine
- ❖ Acid-Base Reaction
  - Calcium salts precipitate in alkaline medium
- ❖ pH Change effects
  - ➢ Solubility
    - Emulsification action of soaps is destroyed in presence of mineral acids
  - ➢ Stability
    - Precipitation of basorin (Active ingredient of Tragacanth) when exposed to pH below 3.0 or above 5.0.
  - ➢ Precipitation
    - Phenobarbital sodium is precipitated as phenobarbaturic acid in lemon syrup
- ❖ Charge Neutralization
  - Anionic Surfactants with Cetrimide
- ❖ Racemization
- ❖ Polymerization
  - Autoclaving dextrose solution turns it into straw colour

THERAPEUTIC

- ❖ Pharmacokinetic
  - ➢ Altered GIT Absorption
    - Altered pH
    - Altered Bacterial Flora
    - Chelation / Complexation
    - Mucosal Damage
    - Altered GIT Motility
  - ➢ Displaced Protein Binding
  - ➢ Altered Metabolism
  - ➢ Altered Renal Excretion
- ❖ Pharmacodynamic Interaction
  - ➢ Additive Effect
  - ➢ Synergistic Effect
  - ➢ Antagonistic Effect

Soap with high concentration in water forms micelles. The overall preparation is transparent.

e.g. *Oil-soluble vitamins A, D are solubilized by polysorbates (non-ionic surfactants)*

2. *Problem*: Concentrated hydroalcoholic solutions of volatile oils, such as spirits (e.g. lemon spirits) and concentrated aromatic water (e.g. concentrated cinnamon water), when used as adjunct (i.e. additive), e.g. as flavoring agents in aqueous preparations.

Consequence: Large globules of oils separate out and and collects as an unsightly (looking bad) surface layer.

Remedy:

(i)   The hydroalcoholic solution should be gradually diluted with the vehicle before mixing with the remaining ingredients.

(ii) The hydroalcoholic solution should be poured slowly into the vehicle with constant stirring.

(iii) Addition of high concentrations of electrolytes (e.g. salts) in which the vehicle is a saturated aqueous solution of a volatile oil.

e.g. *Potassium Citrate Mixture B.P.C. 1973*

Potassium citrate ⟵——— (electrolyte 300............... g)

Citric acid............. 50 g

Lemon spirit.............. 5 ml

Syrup............... 250 ml

Chloroform water D.S............. 300 ml

Water........... 1000 ml

** Quillaia Tincture 1% w/v as emulsifier

When the lemon spirit, used for flavoring, is added the lemon oil is thrown out of the solution, party by the change of solvent and partly by the salting out effect of the high concentration of soluble salt (potassium citrate).

To prevent separation of this oil as surface layer quillaia tincture** is included as an emulsifier.

Insolubility

1. *Problem*: *Liquid preparations containing diffusible solids.*

Consequence: In diffusible solids will produce suspensions those will settle quickly, from which uniform doses cannot be poured out.

Remedy: A thickening agent is necessary to increase the viscosity and reduce the rate of settling of particles.

In diffusible solids

e.g. chalk, aromatic chalk powder, succinyl sulfathiazole and sulphadimidine (in mixture)

e.g. calamine and zinc-oxide (in lotion)

Thickening agents e.g. gum acacia, gum tragacanth, methylcellulose etc.

2. *Problem*: *Wetting problem with insoluble powders.*

   Some insoluble powders like sulphur and certain corticosteroids and antibiotics are difficult to wet with water.

   Consequence: When water is added to such powders a slowly dispersing foam is formed on shaking. This foam is stabilized by fine solid particles.

   Remedy: Wetting agents like saponins or polysorbates are incorporated.

Preparation	Wetting agents used
Sulphur containing lotion	Saponin
Corticosteroid injections	Polysorbate
Antibiotic injections	Polysorbate

3. *Problem*: *Claying of suspensions.*

   When large amount of wetting agents are used, a deflocculated suspension will be produced where all the particles will settle individually and will produce tightly packed sediment. This is called 'claying'.

   Consequence: This tightly packed suspension is difficult to redisperse upon shaking.

   Remedy: Reducing the amount of wetting agent will solve the problem. It will form smaller agglomerates of particles that will settle quickly but will be easily redispersed upon shaking.

4. *Problem*: When a resinous tincture is added to water the water insoluble resin agglomerates forming in diffusible clots.

   Remedy: The undiluted tincture is added slowly to a diluted dispersion of a protective colloid with vigorous stirring.

   e.g. Compound Benzoin tincture

   Benzoin Tincture

   Lobelia Ethereal Tincture

Myrrh Tincture

Tolu Tincture

When these tinctures are diluted with aqueous vehicle the resins precipitate and adheres to the side of the container and forms non-dispersible clots in the liquid. To prevent this the tincture is mixed in a slow stream into the centre of Tragacanth Suspension with rapid stirring.

The hydrocolloids (acacia, tragacanth, and starch) are adsorbed over the surface of the resin particles and confer hydrophilic properties and prevent aggregation into clots.

5. *Problem:* Dispersions of hydrophilic colloids such as acacia or tragacanth mucilage are precipitated by high concentrations of alcohols or salts.

Remedy: Alcohols or salts are well diluted in the vehicle and then the electrolyte or alcohol solution is added slowly into mucilage (hydrophilic colloid) with constant stirring to avoid local high concentration that might neutralize the effect of the protective colloid.

e.g. *Lobelia and Stramonium Mixture, Compound B.P.C.*

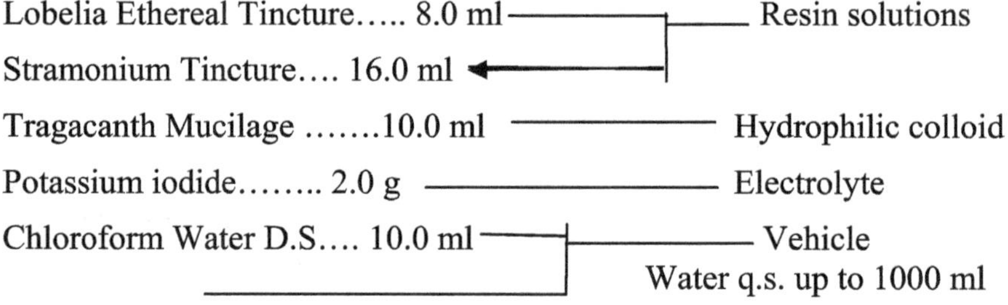

Method – I

1. Half of the vehicle + Tragacanth power

    → Triturated in a mortar and pestle.

    → Tragacanth mucilage is formed.

2. Tincture is poured slowly into the centre of the mucilage with constant stirring.

3. Dissolve the electrolyte into half of the remaining vehicle.

    → Added slowly and stirred to prevent local concentration.

4. The remaining vehicle is added to make up the volume.

Liquefaction

When certain low melting point solids are powdered (triturated in a mortar & pestle) together, a liquid or soft mass is produced due to lowering of melting point of the mixture to below room temperature.

The medicaments those exhibit this type of behaviour are:

(i)   any pair among the following compounds:

camphor, menthol, phenol, thymol, chloral hydrate.

(ii) Sodium salicylate and phenazone

(iii) Aspirin and phenazone

Method-I

If menthol and thymol are required to be dispensed as powder, they are triturated in a mortar to form the liquid mixture. Ingredients that are solids but liquefy on mixing are called Eutectic mixtures. The liquefaction takes place because the melting point of the mixture of these two solids is below the room temperature. the liquid is triturated with enough adsorbent powder e.g. light kaolin or light magnesium carbonate to give a free-flowing product.

N.B. Kaolin and magnesium carbonate are efficient adsorbents and the light category of the powder has a very large specific surface area.

Method-II

If the final bulk volume of powder is very small, then menthol and thymol are triturated separately with small amount of adsorbent powder. Then the two powders are combined lightly and packing the resultant powder in capsules.

The adsorbent powders coat the particles and prevent contact between the medicaments and absorb any liquid that may be produced while triturating.

Chemical Incompatibilities

It is defined as the incompatibility which occurs either due to a chemical reaction or complexation. It can be classified into inorganic or organic type of incompatibilities

Inorganic Incompatibility

General Solubility Principles:

Sodium, Na^+ Potassium, K^+ Ammonium, $NH4^+$	Common Anions	SOLUBLE IN WATER
Chloride, Cl^- Acetate, CH_3COO^- Chlorate, ClO_3^- Nitrate, NO_3^-	Cations of common metals	SOLUBLE IN WATER
Phosphate, PO_4^{3-} Carbonates, CO_3^{2-} Sulphide, S^{2-} Hydroxide, OH^-	Na^+. K^+. NH_4^+.	SOLUBLE IN WATER
Phosphate, PO_4^{3-}. Carbonates, CO_3^{2-}. Sulphide, S^{2-}. Hydroxide, OH^-.	Cations except Na^+, K^+, NH_4^+.	INSOLUBLE IN WATER

Hydrolysis

Salts may hydrolyze to form solutions which may be:

(i) neutral e.g.

$$NaCl \rightleftharpoons \boxed{Na^+ + Cl^-} \longleftarrow \text{Solution is neutral}$$

Strong Electrolyte

(ii) acidic e.g.

$$FeCl_3 + 3H_2O \rightleftharpoons \boxed{Fe(OH)_3 + 3H^+ + 3Cl^-}$$

Solution is acidic

(iii) alkaline e.g.

$$Na_2CO_3 + 2H_2O \rightleftharpoons \boxed{2Na^+ + 2OH^- + H_2CO_3}$$

Solution is alkaline

After hydrolysis the weak base or the weak acid may precipitate out if the amount of the solute is more than its solubility. Hydrolysis occurs to an appreciable extent when one of the products of hydrolysis is insoluble or volatile.

$$FeCl_3 + 3H_2O \rightleftharpoons Fe(OH)_3 + 3HCl .$$

WHY *hydrolysis occurs to an appreciable extent when one of the products of hydrolysis is insoluble or volatile?*

Classification of inorganic incompatibilities:

Metals and their salts	*Group IA*: Sodium (Na), Potassium (K) and Ammonium (NH$_4$) salts
	Group IB: Copper (Cu), Silver (Ag), Gold (Au)
	Group IIA: Magnesium (Mg), Calcium (Ca), Barium (Ba)
	Group IIB: Zinc (Zn), Mercury (Hg)
	Group IIIA: Aluminium (Al)
	Group IVA: Tin (Sn), Lead (Pb)
	Group IVB: Titanium (Ti), Zirconium (Zi)
	Group VA: Arsenic (As), Antimony (Sb), Bismuth (Bi)
	Group VII B: Manganese (Mn)
	Group VIII: Iron (Fe)
Non-metals	Carbon (C), Sulphur (S) and Iodine (I)
Incompatibilities of acids	Strong acids, weak acids, oxidizing acids and reducing acids

Incompatibilities of Metals and their salts

Example of group I alkali metals [Na, K]

Incompatibilities: All the common salts of sodium are soluble in water.

Many sodium salts are soluble in glycerin.

Sodium salts are nearly insoluble in alcohol.

The anionic part of a sodium salt may be precipitated from solution by other metals

Sodium

Sodium bicarbonate (NaHCO$_3$) and Sodium perborate have lowest water solubility among the sodium salts.

Sodium salt	Solubility in water
Sodium bicarbonate	1 in 10
Sodium perborate	1 in 40

So these two sodium salts may precipitate if Na$^+$, HCO^{3-} or perborate ions remain in concentrations above their solubilities in a solution.

Example:

A prescription contains sodium salicylate and potassium bicarbonate.

Incompatibility: Sodium bicarbonate will be formed and precipitated. The solution will darken on standing due to the presence of salicylates in alkaline solution.

$$K^+ \quad + \quad
\begin{array}{c}
COO^- \\
| \\
HO-C-H \\
| \\
HO-C-H \\
| \\
COOH
\end{array}
\quad \longrightarrow \quad
\begin{array}{c}
COOK \\
| \\
HO-C-H \\
| \\
HO-C-H \\
| \\
COOH
\end{array}$$

Precipitate of
Potassium bi tartrate

Potassium

Practically all potassium salts are soluble in water. Only potassium bitartrate (solubility 1 in 165 in water), form precipitates.

Example:

Potassium salts with acidic bitartrate solution

Incompatibility:

Potassium bitartrate will be formed which may precipitate.

Incompatibilities of Non-Metals

Carbon (C)

Activated charcoal

- It is easily oxidized so it is not triturated with oxidizing agents.
- It has adsorptive action hence, it should not be dispensed with potent drugs like alkaloids because the potent drugs will be adsorbed and become inactive.

Sulfur (S)

In pharmacy three forms of powdered-sulfur are available: precipitated, sublimed and washed.

- These powders are soluble only in carbon-disulfide (CS_2) but insoluble in other solvents.

Incompatibilities of Acids

Categories of acids:

1. Strong acid: They are highly ionized in aqueous solution.

   e.g. Perchloric acid ($HClO_4$), sulfuric acid (H_2SO_4), hydrochloric acid (HCl), Hydrobromic acid (HBr), Nitric acid (HNO_3), Phosphoric acid (H_3PO_4)

2. Weak acid: They are slightly ionized in aqueous solution.

   e.g. Acetic acid (CH_3COOH), Carbonic acid (H_2CO_3), hydrogen sulfide (H_2S), hydrocyanic acid (HCN), boric acid (H_3BO_3).

3. Oxidizing acid:

   e.g. Nitric acid (HNO$_3$), Nitric acid + Hydrochloric acid mixture → HCl + HNO$_3$ + NOCl + Cl$_2$.

   Permanganic acid (KMNO$_4$), Chromic acid (H$_2$CrO$_4$), Perboric acid (HBO$_3$) and Nitrous acid (HNO$_2$)

4. Reducing acid:

   e.g. Hypo phosphorous acid (H$_3$PO$_2$), sulfuric acid (H$_2$SO$_3$), hydroiodic acid (HI), thiosulfuric acid (H$_2$SO$_3$), thiocyanic acid (HSCN).

Nitric acid (HNO$_3$) *Oxidizing acid*

   (i)   HNO$_3$ reacts with some alkaloids to form colored compounds.

   (ii) It forms explosive nitroglycerin when rotated with sulfuric acid and glycerin.

   (iii) Fe^{++}, arsenous and mercurous salts are oxidized by HNO$_3$ into their oxidized state.

   (iv) Nitrates (like KNO$_3$) + Charcoal

   (v)   chemicals such as sulfur, sucrose and glycerin are also not compatible with Nitric acid

Hypochlorous acid (HOCl) (*Reducing acid*)

HOCl is unstable.

Hypochlorites (e.g. Sodium hypochlorite, NaOCl) are decomposed by acids, even H$_2$CO$_3$ with the liberation of unstable HOCl. Solutions of hypochlorites must be prepared at room temperature, because heat converts them into chlorates and chlorides.

Hydrogen peroxide (H$_2$O$_2$)

Hydrogen peroxide decomposes slowly with the evolution of oxygen. Heat increases the role of reaction.

Hydroiodic acid (HI) (Reducing acid)

HI and I$^-$ in acidic solution turn brown on standing, free iodine being released.

$$2HI \rightarrow H_2 + I_2.$$

$$4\,I^- + O_2 + 2H^+ \rightarrow 2\,I_2 + 2H_2O$$

Examples of acid preparation

Fluid extract: Ergot, ipecac, nux vomica, aconite.

Elixir: Compound pepsin, compound glycero phosphates, lactated pepsin.

Solutions: Ammonium acetate, ferric chloride, iron and ammonium acetate, ferrous sulfate, Hydrogen peroxide, magnesium citrate.

Syrups: Citric acid, hydroiodic acid, cherry, ferrous iodide, orange, raspberry, squill, ipecac.

Glycerites: boroglycerin, pepsin

Tinctures: aconite, ferric chloride, camphorated opium, nux vomica, cinchona.

Miscellaneous: Squill vinegar

Preparations having an alkaline reaction

They have general incompatibilities of alkalies:

e.g. (i)   neutralization of acids,

(ii)   precipitation of alkaloids

(iii)   precipitation

(iv)   liberation of NH_3 from ammonium salts.

Alkaline preparation

Fluid extract: Senega

Ointments: Rose water

Solutions: lead subacetate, sodium hypochlorite, $Ca(OH)_2$, soda and mint.

Spirits: aromatic ammonia

Syrups: senega, ginger, rhubarb

Water: Ammonia

General Organic Incompatibilities

1. Hydrocarbons:

They include both saturated and unsaturated compounds of C and H.

- Over exposure to volatile hydrocarbons may cause damage to the heart, liver or kidneys.

- A hydrocarbon may produce Vitamin A, D, E and K deficiency on prolonged use or exposure.

(a) Saturated hydrocarbon

Saturated hydrocarbons used in pharmacy include:

Petroleum ether $(C_5 - C_7)$

Deodorized kerosene ($C_9 - C_{15}$)

Light mineral oil ($C_{15} - C_{20}$)

Mineral oil ($C_{18} - C_{24}$)

Petrolatum ($C_{18} - C_{30}$),   White petrolatum ($C_{18} - C_{30}$)

Paraffin ($C_{24} - C_{30}$).

Sometimes unsaturated hydrocarbons may remain as impurities, which may degrade to produce rancidity. So dl-α-tocopherol (another name is Vit. E) is used as antioxidant.

(b) Unsaturated hydrocarbons

Contains double bonds (called *alkenes*), or triple bond(s) (called *alkynes*).

Reactions of unsaturated hydrocarbons:

(i)   addition type reactions : unsaturated bonds may add Br_2, HBr, H_2, H_2SO_4)

(ii)   may be oxidized at unsaturation point

(iii) may be reduced at the unsaturation point.

(c) Aromatic hydrocarbon

Benzene, naphthalene, anthracene – these are not found in prescription.

(d) Hydrogenated hydrocarbons

e.g. Chloroform ($CHCl_3$), ethyl bromide (C_2H_5Br) etc.

They are immiscible with water, soluble in alcohol and organic solvents.

(e) Alcohols

$$C_2H_5OH + HI \longrightarrow C_2H_5I + H_2O$$

(Ethanol)   (Ethyl iodide)

- Ethanol and methanol are incompatible with acacia, albumins and oxidizing agents such as chlorine, bromine, permanganate and chromic acid.

Purine bases:

e.g.   Caffeine (1,3,7 trimethyl xanthine)

         theobromine (3,7 dimethyl xanthine)

         theophylline (1,3 dimethyl xanthine)

Purine

Xanthine derivative

Properties:

They are very weak bases and cannot form salts with acid also.

Alkaloids

Solubility

Solvent	Free alkaloids	Alkaloidal salts
Water	No	Yes
Ether	Yes	No
Chloroform	Yes	No
Oils	Yes	No

Reactions

Reactants	Free alkaloids	Alkaloidal salts
Alkaline reactants 　Borax 　Sodium phosphate 　Potassium citrate		Precipitation of insoluble free alkaloids
Tannins	Precipitation of tannates	Precipitation
Organic acids	Precipitation	Precipitation
Picric acid Iodine Potassium iodide Potassium mercuric iodide Mercuric chloride Gold chloride	Precipitation	Precipitation

General remedies

1. In low concentration the alkaloid may not precipitate out of the solution, because the free alkaloid may also have slight solubility.

2. In many cases this problem may be solved by adding alcohol, because free alkaloidal bases are soluble in alcoholic solution.

3. If there is a possibility of precipitation, then it is advisable to display the message "*Shake the bottle before use*" on the label.

4. In some cases, it is feasible to add some acacia mucilage or other suspending agent to retard the settling of the precipitate.

5. Aqueous solutions of alkaloidal salts frequently show a precipitate due to mold growth. Chlorobutanol (0.5%) may be incorporated as preservative.

Examples of incompatibilities

1. *Alkaloidal salts with soluble iodides*

    Alkaloidal salts will react with soluble iodides and may precipitate insoluble iodide salts of alkaloids.

Alklaoidal salts	Soluble iodide
Emetine hydrochloride Methadome hydrochloride Strychnine hydrochloride Papaverine hydrochloride	Potassium iodide

Incompatibility

Emetine-HCl + KI $\rightarrow$ Emetine-HI + KCl

Solubility of Emetine-HI is less hence may precipitate.

Example: Potassium iodide is used as expectorant in some alkaloid containing cough mixtures.

Remedy: If the alkaloid concentration is very low then precipitation does not occur.

2. *Alkaloidal salts with tannins*

    Incompatibility:

    Alkaloidal salts + tannins $\rightarrow$ Alkaloidal tannates$\downarrow$

    N.B. One advantage of this reaction is in case of alkaloidal poisoning. strong tea (or tannic acid solution) is used to precipitate the alkaloids.

    Remedy: Method-B (suspended with the help of tragacanth mucilage) is used to suspend the precipitate.

Pyrazolon derivatives

e.g. Antipyrine, aminopyrine are non-narcotic analgesic

Incompatibilities

1. They produce color when mixed with oxidizing agents.

2. The solid compounds have a tendency to liquefy or form a soft mass when triturated with a number of hydrogen-bonding substances.

Aliphatic amino acids and derivatives

Amino acids are carboxylic acids which contain an amino (NH_2) group attached to any carbon atom in the radical attached to carboxyl.

e.g.

$$H_2N\;\underset{\underset{R}{|}}{CH}\;COOH$$

Solubility: Soluble in water, insoluble in alcohol.

They are amphoteric, forming either hydrochloride or sodium salts.

Examples of aliphatic amino acids: amino acetic acid, methionine.

Quaternary ammonium compounds

These compounds have the general formula of

R_4NX

where   R = alkyl or aryl group

X = Cl, OH

e.g.   Trimethylammonium chloride, $(CH_3)_4N^+Cl^-$

Incompatibilities:

1. Quaternary ammonium bases are very soluble in water and readily absorb carbon dioxide from air.

2. These are highly ionized and react with the anions of weak acids (e.g fatty acids, acidic dyes, certain antibiotics, and barbiturates) to form insoluble complexes, e.g.

$$(R4N)^+Cl^- \;+\; Na^+\;{}^-OOC\,R \;\rightleftharpoons\; RCOONR_4 \;+\; Na^+ \;+\; Cl^-$$

| Benzalkonium chloride | Sodium stearate | Benzalkonium stearate |

Thus, efficacy of quaternary ammonium germicides reduces in presence of alkali soaps or other anionic surfactants.

Remedy: The addition of inorganic or organic salts (e.g. NaCl) will solubilize such complexes.

Therapeutic Incompatibility

Usually this incompatibility arises when one or more drugs produce response or intensity different from that intended in the patients.

Classification

Over doses

Under doses

Improper consumption by the patient

Contra-indicated drugs

A. Over doses: This can be sub grouped as follows:

Excessive single dose

Sometimes a single dose may become overdose depending on the health of the patient e.g. a normal dose (taking body weight as 70 kg for an adult male) may be overdose for a lowly built person. However, it should not be more than 2 to 3 normal dose.

Remedy: The pharmacist should consult the physician and clarify the dose.

e.g. 1   Rx

Atropine sulphate	6 mg
Phenobarbital	360 mg

Make capsules.

Label: One capsule to be taken three times a day before meals.

Comments: In this prescription the doses of both atropine sulphate and phenobarbital are 12 times the normal doses. The physician intended for 12 capsules to be dispensed but he has mistaken or maybe it is an incomplete prescription. Hence, before dispensing the pharmacist should consult the physician again.

Correct prescription

Rx

Atropine sulphate	6 mg
Phenobarbital	360 mg

Make capsules. Supply 12 capsules.

Label: One capsule to be taken three times a day before meals.

e.g. 2   Rx

Strychnine sulphate	20 mg
Iron and ammonium citrate	500 mg

Prepare capsules. Supply 12 capsules.

Label: One capsule to be taken three times a day after meals.

Comment: 10 times overdose of strychnine hydrochloride than that of normal. The pharmacist should consult the physician and obtain the permission to change the dose.

Corrected prescription

Strychnine sulphate	2 mg
Iron and ammonium citrate	500 mg

Prepare capsules. Supply 12 capsules.

Label: One capsule to be taken three times a day after meals.

Excessive daily dose

In this case the daily dose of drug is exceeded.

e.g.1   Rx

Codeine phosphate	15 mg
Ammonium chloride	500 mg

Prepare capsules and supply 24 capsules.

Label: Two capsules to be taken every hour for cough.

Comment: The U.S.P. recommends that the prescribed dose should be taken after every four hours and not every hour. Hence the physician should be consulted.

Additive and synergistic combinations:

There are certain drugs possessing similar pharmacological activity. If these drugs are combined together, they may produce additive or synergistic action. In such case advice of the physician is necessary.

e.g.   Rx

Amphetamine sulphate	20 mg
Ephedrine sulphate	50 mg
Syrup q.s.	100 ml

Let a mixture be made

Label: Take 25 ml every four hours.

Comment: Both the drugs are sympathetic stimulants and they are prescribed in their full dose. The formulation will produce additive overdose effect. Hence, the dose of individual drug should be reduced.

B. Under dose: In this type of incompatibility, effect of one drug is reduced or antagonise by the presence of another drug. This can be exemplified by combination of following types of drugs:

Stimulants like nux-vomica, strychnine sulphate, caffeine etc. with **sedatives** like barbiturates, paraldehyde etc.

Sympathomimetic or **adrenergic** like ephedrine, nor-adrenaline with **sympatholytic** drugs like ergotamine.

Sympathetic stimulants like methamphetamine with **parasympathetic stimulants** like pilocarpine.

Purgatives like castor oil, liquid paraffin etc with **antidiarrheal** agents like bismuth carbonates.

Acidifiers like dilute hydrochloric acid and **alkalisers** like sodium bicarbonate, magnesium carbonate.

Comment: In all the cases the pharmacist should consult with the doctor who had prescribed it and one drug should be removed from the prescription.

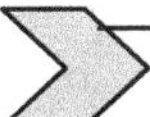

Practical Based on Incompatibilities

1. AIM- To prepare insufflation powder I.P. (100mg) (Physical Incompatibility) (LIQUIFACTION)

Ingredients	Qty prescribed
Menthol	5 mg
Camphor	5 mg
Ammonium Chloride	30 mg
Light magnesium Carbonate	60 mg

Theory: Incompatibility is a condition which arises when two or more ingredients on mixing interact in such a way that their properties get altered. Physical incompatibility is a condition which arises when ingredients on mixing react to produce precipitates, evolve gases like carbon dioxide or undergo other physical changes. Insufflations are medicated dusting powders that are intended for application to nasal cavity. The drugs which get destroyed in gastrointestinal tract can be administered through this way. Insufflation powder containing menthol, camphor, ammonium chloride and light magnesium carbonate is used for treating various nasal infections where physical compatibility arises on mixing the active ingredients such as camphor and menthol which on mixing form eutectic mixture i.e. become liquid. To overcome this problem, it is triturated with a known amount of light magnesium carbonate which act as an adsorbent and helps in formation of solid dosage form that can be easily administered. Ammonium Chloride present in prescription acts as deliquescent (absorbs moisture from air and hence prevents the drying up of tissue).

Procedure: Mix methanol and camphor. Then add known amount of light magnesium carbonate with trituration until the liquid mixture converts into solid. Finally add Ammonium chloride to the mixture, triturate and finally dispense in doubly wrapped paper.

Uses: Used for treating blocked nose and administrating drugs for nasal cavity.

Precautions-Do not swallow.

2. **AIM- To prepare sodium salicylate and caffeine solution I.P. (30ml).**

    (Chemical incompatibility- Adjusted chemical incompatibility)

Ingredients	Quantity prescribed	Remedial Formula	Quantity Prescribed
Sodium Salicylate	1.00g	Sodium Salicylate	1.00g
Caffeine Citrate	0.65g	Caffeine	0.325g
Purified water q.s.	30.000ml	Purified water q.s.	30.000ml

Theory: Sodium salicylate and caffeine citrate is an example of *adjusted chemical incompatibility,* where the interaction between the ingredients is minimized by replacing one or more ingredients without affecting its overall therapeutic value. A solution of salicylate with alkaloid salts such as sodium salicylate with caffeine citrate leads to formation of salicylic acid. Caffeine citrate on interaction with water yields citrate ion which provides acidic conditions and converts salicylate ion into salicylic acid which irritates the gastric mucosa causing ulcers and pain. Hence to prevent the formation of caffeine citrate, it is replaced with half amount of caffeine as both are equipotent in nature and caffeine does not enable the formation of salicylic acid.

Remedy: Use Caffeine roughly ½ weight of caffeine citrate.

Procedure: Dissolve caffeine and sodium salicylate in sufficient amount of water to produce the required volume.

Uses: Analgesic, CNS Stimulant, Treatment of Migraine, Draught

3. **AIM- To prepare caffeine citrate and aromatic spirit of ammonia solution I.P. (30ml).**

    Incompatibility between alkaloidal salt and alkaline substance (Tolerated chemical incompatibility) (DIFFISIBLE PRECIPITATES)

Ingredients	Qty prescribed
Caffeine citrate	0.65g
Aromatic spirit of ammonia	4.00ml
Purified water q.s.	120.00ml

Theory: A solution of caffeine citrate and aromatic spirit of ammonia is an example of chemical incompatibility due to formation of diffusible precipitates of alkaloid salts in basic medium.

Remedy: (Method A) Dissolve caffeine citrate in water in one beaker and mix aromatic spirit of ammonia in water in another beaker and then add solution of aromatic spirit of ammonia drop wise to the caffeine citrate solution.

Uses: Respiratory Stimulant (decreases fatigue by increasing oxygen consumption).

4. **AIM – To prepare quinine Hydrochloride Sodium Salicylate Solution**

Ingredients	Qty prescribed	Remedial Ingredients	Qty prescribed
Quinine HCl	1.20 g	Quinine HCl	1.20 g
Sod. Salicylate	4.00 g	Sod. Salicylate	4.00 g
Purified Water q.s.	100.00 g	Compound powder of Tragacanth	2.00 g
		Purified water q.s.	100.0 ml

Theory: This prescription shows chemical incompatibility, because quinine hydrochloride is an alkaloidal salt, which reacts with sodium salicylate, and precipitate quinine salicylate. This precipitation is in diffusible in nature.

Remedy: (METHOD B) – A suspending agent (Compound powder of tragacanth) 2 gm/ 100 ml is used to suspend the resulting precipitant.

Procedure: Separately weight sodium salicylate and compound powder of tragacanth and transfer into mortar and triturate them properly. Weigh quinine hydrochloride and dissolve in water and add this solution to the mortar and mix well by trituration. Transfer the prepared mixture to a measuring cylinder, and after rinsing the residue from mortar to measuring cylinder make up the volume and mix them well.

Dispensing: Store in amber colored bottle as quinine is sensitive to light

USES: Anti-Malarial, analgesic.

Direction: One tablespoonful after meals

Storage: Store in cool place

Auxiliary Label: SHAKE THE BOTTLE WELL BEFORE USE

5. **Prepare sodium salicylate and sodium bicarbonate solution I.P. (30ml).**

    (Incompatibility of soluble salicylate with alkali bicarbonates) (Oxidative Color Change)

Ingredients	Quantity	Remedial Formula	Quantity
Sodium Salicylate	1.00g	Sodium Salicylate	1.00g
Sodium Bicarbonate	1.00g	Sodium Bicarbonate	1.00g
Chloroform water q.s.	15.00ml	Sodium metabisulphite	0.01g
		Chloroform water q.s.	15.00ml

Theory: A solution of sodium salicylate with sodium bicarbonate solution is an example of adjusted chemical incompatibility where the interaction between the ingredients is minimized without affecting the overall composition of the formulation. Sodium bicarbonate presents in the formulation prevent the precipitation of salicylic acid on exposure to acidic conditions of stomach by neutralizing the acid present in it. However, sodium bicarbonate provides alkaline medium to sodium salicylate, due to which sodium salicylate absorbs oxygen from air and form an oxidized product, which turns the solution reddish brown in color. Hence, the formulation acquires reddish brown color on storage. However, there is no effect on its therapeutic value. To prevent this, a small amount of coloring agent/ antioxidants like sodium metabisulphite is added.

Remedy-Add antioxidant like sodium metabisulphite approx 0.01g per 15ml of preparation.

Procedure: Dissolve sodium salicylate, sodium bicarbonate and sodium metabisulphite in sufficient amount of chloroform water to produce 30ml.

Use: Analgesic.

6.   **AIM- To prepare sodium salicylate and ferric chloride solution.**

   Incompatibility between soluble salicylate with ferric salts (INDIFFUSIBLE PRECIPITATES)

Ingredients	Qty prescribed	Remedial Formula	Qty
Sodium Salicylate	4.00g	Sodium Salicylate	4.00g
Ferric Chloride Solution	2.00ml	Sodium Bicarbonate	4.00g
Purified water q.s.	100.00ml	Ferric Chloride Solution	2.00ml
		Purified water q.s.	100.00ml

Theory: A Solution of sodium salicylate with ferric chloride solution is a case of incompatibility where there is formation of in diffusible precipitate of ferric salicylate by reaction between ferric chloride and sodium salicylate. The precipitate is in diffusible in neutral medium hence, the therapeutic value of the formulation decreases. To prevent this, a small amount of sodium bicarbonate is added which provides alkaline medium.

Procedure: Dissolve sodium salicylate and sodium bicarbonate in 10ml of water. Then add ferric chloride solution to the above solution and finally add sufficient water to produce the required volume.

Uses: Iron supplement, treating anemia, Hemorrhage (Ferric chloride is an astringent)

7. **AIM- To prepare Sodium Metaborate solution I.P. (30 ml).**

    Incompatibility due to evaluation of gas

Ingredients	Qty prescribed
Sodium Bicarbonate	1.50 g
Borax	1.50 ml
Phenol	0.75 g
Glycerin	25.00 g
Purified water q.s.	100.00 ml

Theory: In the formulation containing borax glycerin, sodium bicarbonate, phenol, and water, borax hydrolysis to yield boric acid which react with glycerin to produce glyceroboric acid. The later further reacts with sodium bicarbonate forming sodium metaborate and glycerin with evolution of carbon dioxide. The evolution of carbon dioxide is slow, which is hastened by using hot water. To prevent leakage or explosion, the reaction must be completed before the preparation is bottled and thus it is carried out in an open vessel.

Reaction–$Na_2B_4O_7.10H_2O + H_2O \rightarrow 2H_3BO_3$(Boric Acid) + $NaBO_2$ (Sodium Metaborate) (Borax)

Boric Acid + Glycerol $\rightarrow$ Glyceroboric Acid

Glyceroboric acid + $NaHCO_3 \rightarrow$ Sodium Metaborate + Glycerin + CO_2 (gas)

Procedure: Mix all the ingredients in an open vessel using hot water as the vehicle till the evolution of gas cease. Then dispense the formulation.

Uses: Topical antiseptic

8. **AIM- To prepare Sodium Citrate, Magnesium citrate solution (30 ml) Incompatibility due to evolution of gas**

Ingredients	Qty prescribed
Magnesium Carbonate	1.0 g
Sodium Bicarbonate	1.0 g
Citric acid	1.0 g
Purified water q.s.	60.0 ml

Theory: Magnesium carbonate is insoluble and will react with citric acid to from magnesium citrate in solution. Sodium bicarbonate is soluble in liquid. If citric acid is dissolved first in water and then sodium bicarbonates added to this solution, followed by magnesium carbonate, a clear and complete solution is not produced, since some of the magnesium carbonate will remain unchanged.

Citric Acid + Sodium Bicarbonate →Sodium Citrate

Sodium Citrate + Magnesium Carbonate →Magnesium carbonate remains as suspension

Magnesium Carbonate + Citric Acid → Magnesium Citrate + CO_2↑

On the other hand, a perfectly clean solution can be obtained by adding the magnesium carbonate to the solution of citric acid first. Then allow these two compounds to react completely to form solution of magnesium citrate and then adding the sodium bicarbonate. The reason for this order of mixing is that both magnesium carbonate and sodium bicarbonate will react with citric acid in solution. When bicarbonate ion is added first it uses some of citric acid so that not enough is left to convert all the magnesium carbonate to solubilize magnesium citrate. As a result, the carbonate that is left will not dissolve by reacting the magnesium carbonate and citric acid. First, all of the carbonate is converted to the citrate then the sodium bicarbonate which is water soluble is added to give a clean solution.

Procedure: Dissolve sodium bicarbonate and citric acid in one part of water in an open vessel. In another part of water dissolve magnesium carbonate. Then mix the two solutions slowly with constant stirring. When the evolution of gas ceases, dispense the formulation.

Use: Antacid.

9. **AIM- To prepare Magnesium Carbonate suspension counter incompatibility due to evolution of gas (30 ml).**

Ingredients	Qty prescribed
Magnesium sulphate	16.0 g
Sodium Bicarbonate	8.0 g
Peppermint water q.s.	120.0 ml

Theory: Magnesium sulphate and sodium bicarbonate react resulting in a double decomposition where there is formation of magnesium bicarbonate which decomposes forming insoluble carbonate and carbon dioxide.

$$MgSO_4 + 2NaHCO_3 \rightarrow Na_2SO_4 + Mg(HCO_3)_2$$

$$Mg(HCO_3)_2 \rightarrow MgCO_3 (↓) + H_2O + CO2 \text{ (gas) } ↑$$

The evolution of carbon dioxide is an endothermic reaction which is hastened by using hot water and the reaction is carried out in open vessel to prevent leakage or explosion. Moreover, the magnesium carbonate precipitate is diffusible in nature so it is diluted with one part of water and then mixed with other reactant dissolved in another part of vehicle. Peppermint water in the prescription is used as a flavored vehicle, which is used as such without heating it because if it is heated, then it will result in loss of aroma of volatile ingredient present in it.

Procedure: Dissolve magnesium sulphate in 10 ml of hot water. Dissolve sodium bicarbonate in another 10 ml of hot water and add slowly to magnesium sulphate with constant stirring. Then add sufficient peppermint water to produce the required volume to 30 ml and dispense it.

Uses: Magnesium supplement, Antacid

Auxiliary Label: Shake well before use.

10. AIM- To Prepare Phenol Zinc Oxide Solution (30 ml)

Counter incompatibility due to formation of complex

Ingredients	Qty prescribed	Remedial Ingredients	Qty prescribed
Phenol	1.00 g	Phenol	1.00 g
Zinc Oxide	15.00 g	Zinc Oxide	15.00 g
PEG-200	10.00 g	Bentonite	10.00 g
Purified water q.s.	100.0 ml	Purified water q.s.	100.0 ml

Theory– In this preparation, incompatibility mainly arises due to formation of complex due to interaction of polyethylene glycol-200 (PEG-200) with phenol. The -OH group of phenol undergoes hydrogen bonding with oxygen atom of PEG-200 resulting in formation of a complex which settles down and separates as an elegant product. The formation of complex leads to inactivation of the drug as the active ingredient is present inside the polymer. Thus, to keep the therapeutic value intact, PEG-200 to replaced with bentonite which functions as a suspending agent and thickener and prevent the inactivation of the drug keeping its pharmacological value intact and increasing its shelf life.

Procedure: Triturate zinc oxide and bentonite in mortar and pestle with a small quantity of water until a smooth paste is formed. Dissolve phenol in water and add to zinc oxide solution slowly with constant stirring until a smooth solution is formed. Add sufficient water to produce required volume and dispense.

Uses: Antimicrobial, Antiseptic, for treating psoriasis.

Unit 5

Semisolid Dosage Forms

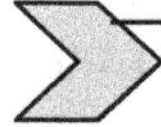

Definition

Pharmaceutical semisolid dosage preparations include ointments, pastes, cream, emulsions, gels and rigid foams.

Ointments are soft semisolid preparations meant for external application to the skin or mucous membrane. They usually contain medicament, which is either dissolved or suspended in the base.

They have emollient and protective action.

Creams are semisolid emulsions for external application and are generally of softer consistency and lighter than ointments.

They are less greasy and are easy to apply.

Pastes are semisolid preparations for external application that differs from similar products in containing a high proportion of finely powdered medicaments. They are stiffer and are usually employed for their protective action and for their ability to absorb serous discharges from skin lesions.

Thus, when protective, rather than therapeutic action is desired, the formulation pharmacists will favor a paste, but when therapeutic action is required, he will prefer ointments and creams.

Jellies are transparent or translucent, non-greasy, semisolid preparation mainly used externally.

In these systems the liquid phase is entrapped within a three-dimensional polymeric matrix in which a high degree of physical cross-linking has been introduced.

The polymers (gelling agents) used include:

Natural Polymers: Tragacanth, pectin, carrageenan, agar, alginic acid and gelatin.

Synthetic and Semisynthetic polymers: Methyl cellulose, hydroxymethyl cellulose, carboxymethyl cellulose and Carbopols.

Structure of Skin

The skin has three main layers: the epidermis, dermis and hypodermis.

Epidermis is the outermost layer. It consists of:

(a) The *basal layer* (innermost) is one cell thick layer. Its cells divide constantly and the daughter cells are steadily pushed towards the surface.

(b) The *prickle cell layer*: The cells in this region are linked by tiny bridges or prickles.

(c) The *granular layer*: When they reach this region, the upwardly moving cells become granules and begin to synthesize the inert protein keratin.

(d) The *horny layer* (stratum corneum). This is the outermost layer and the cells are heavily keratinized and dead. The dead cells slough off gradually.

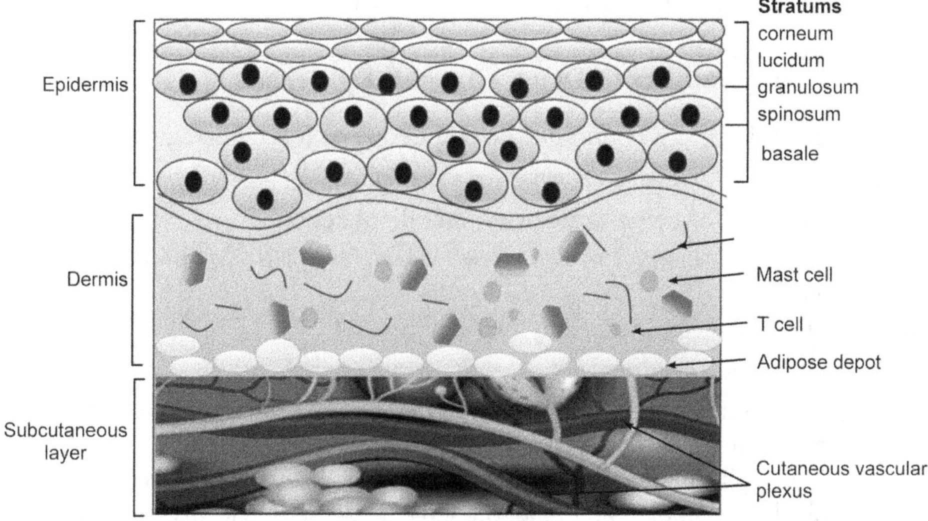

Structure of Skin

Dermis is the middle and the main part of the skin. The dermis is made up of protein collagen and elastin. The collagen is in the form of gel that is reinforced by a framework of elastin.

Dermis contains the following structures:

(a) Blood vessels, lymphatics and nerves.

(b) Epidermal appendages e.g. hair follicles, sebaceous glands and sweat glands.

Hypodermis, the innermost layer, consists of adipose tissues. It gives physical protection and thermal insulation to underlying structures.

(N.B. Epidermis is non-granular but is penetrated by hair follicles, sebaceous glands and sweat glands.

Sebum is the secretion of sebaceous glands, which is a mixture of fatty substances and emulsifiers; it mixes with water producing a fluid of pH 5.5 that covers the skin surface and permeates the upper layer of keratinized cells – this is called the *"acid-mantle"* of skin.

Keratin is hydrophillic, the stratum corneum normally contains about 20% w/w of water, the amount varying with atmospheric humidity. This moisture keeps the skin supple and if its level falls below about 12% the cells becomes dry and brittle and then shrink and curl at the edges, making the skin feel rough.

Cracking may cause discomfort. Loss of water may be the result of excessive evaporation, over-usage of detergents (which removes sebum) and cold weather (which inhibits sebum production).

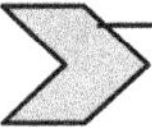 ## Permeability of Drug Through Epidermis

Most dermatological preparations belong to one of following classes:

1. *Preparation intended to remain on the surface*

   e.g. products for penetration or for emollient action.

2. *Preparations intended to penetrate the skin but will not enter into blood stream*

Drugs penetrate the epidermis by two-man routes:

(a) *Through the keratinized cells of the stratum corneum.*

   The keratinized cells are fused together so drug molecules directly diffuse through them. These cells contain keratin which is hydrophilic and phospholipids which is hydrophobic, so drug molecules having solubility in both water and oil have good permeability through this route.

(b) *Via hair follicles*

   Although the hair follicles occupy only a small area of the total epidermis, they provide a very important route of penetration. The fat-soluble drugs dissolve in sebum, diffuses in to the sebum-filled follicles and passes to dermis.

Factor Affecting Permeability of a Drug Through Skin

A.   Factor associated with the skin

(a) *Hydration of the horny layer*

   The hydration of keratinized cells is raised by covering the area with a moisture-proof plastic film to prevent evaporation of perspiration. Hydration increases the drug penetration.

(b) *Thickness of the horny layer*

The horny layer is thickest on palms and soles and thinnest on the face; penetration rate increases with decreased thickness of horny layer.

(c) *Skin condition*

The permeability of the skin is affected by age, disease, climate and injury. For example, absorption occurs rapidly in children and if the dermis is exposed by a wound or burn.

B.   Factors associated with the medicament

(a) *Solubility of the drug*

Highly lipid soluble molecules enter through hair follicles. Moderately lipid soluble molecules penetrate directly across the horny layer.

(b) *Dissociation constant (pK$_a$)*

If a drug is ionized in the surrounding pH of the dermis, then the penetration of the ionic species is restricted by electrostatic interactions. Degree of ionization depends on the pK$_a$ of the drug.

e.g. Methyl salicylate and methyl nicotinate penetrate much faster than salicylic acid and nicotinic acid respectively.

(c) *Particle size*

Reducing the particle size increases, the dissolution of a poorly soluble drug in suspension and thus increases the release rate from the vehicle.

(d) *Crystal structure*

The metastable polymorph is much more soluble than its stable form, so the release of drug in metastable state is much faster than stable form.

C.   Factors associated with vehicles

The rate of release of a drug from a vehicle to stratum corneum is governed by *vehicle-to-stratum corneum partition coefficient*. The thermodynamic activity of the drug in the vehicle is the product of the concentration of the drug and the activity coefficient (γ) of the drug in the vehicle. Drugs held firmly by the vehicle exhibit low activity coefficient, release from the drug-vehicle combination is slow. Drug held loosely by the vehicle shows higher activity coefficient, hence shows faster rate of release.

The vehicles may enhance the penetration of a drug in one or more of the following ways:

✓ By ensuring good contact with the surface of the body

✓ By increasing the degree of hydration of the stratum corneum

✓ By penetrating the epidermis

✓ By directly altering the permeability of the skin

(a) *Contact with body surface*

Sticky bases such as soft paraffin, Paraffin ointment B.P.C., Simple ointment B.P. etc. adheres well to the skin but are difficult to apply evenly and remove completely.

Creams are easier to apply and remove. Oil in water (o/w) creams mix with sebum and are more suitable for weeping or wounded surface.

(b) *Hydration of stratum corneum*

An occlusive layer reduces evaporation of water from skin, increasing hydration of the horny layer and, therefore, promotes penetration of medicament.

e.g. hydrocarbons, wool fat and isopropyl myristate containing ointments produce occlusive films on the skin. Water in oil (o/w) type creams have some occlusive effects.

Humectants like glycerol's are not good for retaining water because at low atmospheric humidities, because they tend to increase loss of water by absorbing it from the skin.

(c) *Penetration of the epidermis*

Bases miscible with the sebum penetrate into the regions of the skin in which sebum is found.

e.g. Wool fat (originating from sebaceous glands of sheep) penetrates into the skin.

Vegetable oils penetrate more slowly and liquid paraffin does not penetrate at all.

(d) *Alteration of skin permeability*

Penetration can be improved by dissolving the medicament in an organic liquid such as ethanol, dimethylformamide (DMF), dimethyl acetamide, dimethyl sulfoxide (DMSO) and propylene glycol. They increase the hydration of skin.

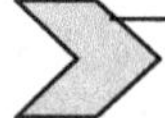 **Ointments**

Ointments are semisolid preparations for application to the skin or mucosae. The ointment bases are almost always anhydrous and generally contain one or more medicaments in suspension or solution.

Characteristics of an ideal ointment:

It should be chemically and physically stable.

It should be smooth and free from grittiness.

It should melt or soften at body temperature and be easily applied.

The base should be non-irritant and should have no therapeutic action.

The medicament should be finely divided and uniformly distributed throughout the base.

Classification of ointments

According to their therapeutic properties based on penetration of skin.

According to their therapeutic uses.

Ointments classified according to their therapeutic properties based on penetration are as follows:

(a)   Epidermic, (b) Endodermic, (c) Diadermic

(a)   Epidermic ointments

These ointments are intended to produce their action on the surface of the skin and produce local effect.

They are not absorbed.

They act as protectives, antiseptics and parasiticides.

(b)   Endodermic ointments

These ointments are intended to release the medicaments that penetrate into the skin. They are partially absorbed and acts as emollients, stimulants and local irritants.

(c)   Diadermic ointments

These ointments are intended to release the medicaments that pass through the skin and produce systemic effects.

According to therapeutic uses the ointments are classified as follows:

1.	Acne treatment	resorcinol, sulfur
2.	Antibiotics	Used to kill microorganisms. e.g. bacitracin, chlortetracycline, neomycin
3.	Anti-inflammatory	Used to relieve inflammatory, allergic and pruritic conditions of the skin. e.g. betamethasone valerate, hydrocortisone, triamcinolone acetonide
4.	Ant eczematous	Used to stop oozing and exudation from vesicles on the skin. e.g. hydrocortisone, coal tar, ichthammol, salicylic acid.
5.	Antifungal	Used to inhibit or kill the fungi. e.g. benzoic acid, salicylic acid, nystatin, clotrimazole, etc
6.	Antipruritic	Used to relieve itching. e.g. benzocaine, coal tar.
7.	Antiseptic	Used to stop sepsis. e.g. ammoniated mercury, zinc oxide.
8.	Astringent	Reduces the secretion of glands or discharge from skin surface. e.g. calamine, zinc oxide, aluminium acetate and subacetate, acetic acid and tannic acid.

Contd...

9	Counter irritant	These are applied locally to irritate the intact skin, thus reducing or relieving another irritation or deep-seated pain. e.g. capsicum oleoresin, iodine (Iodex), methyl salicylate.
10.	Dandruff treatment	e.g. salicylic acid and cetrimide (cetyl trimethyl ammonium bromide)
11.	Emollient	Used to soften the skin (for example in the dry season). e.g. soft paraffin
12.	Keratolytic	Used to remove or soften the horny layer of the skin. e.g. resorcinol, salicylic acid and sulfur.
13.	Keratoplastic	Tends to increase the thickness of horny layer e.g. coal tar.
14.	Parasiticide	These ointments destroy or inhibit living infestations such as lice and ticks. e.g. benzyl benzoate, gamma-benzene hexachloride (GBH), sulfur
15.	Protective	Protects the skin from moisture, air, sun rays or other substances such as soaps or chemicals. e.g. silicones, titanium dioxide, calamine, zinc oxide, petrolatum.

Ointment Bases

The ointment base is that substance or part of an ointment preparation which serves as carrier or vehicle for the medicament.

An ideal ointment base should be inert, stable, smooth, compatible with the skin, non-irritating and should release the incorporated medicaments readily.

Classification of ointment bases:

1. Oleaginous bases
2. Absorption bases
3. Water-miscible bases
4. Water soluble bases

Oleaginous Bases

These bases consist of oils and fats. The most important are:

Hydrocarbons i.e. petrolatum, paraffins and mineral oils.

The *animal fat* includes lard.

The combination of these materials can produce a product of desired melting point and viscosity.

(a) Petrolatum (Soft paraffin)

This is a purified mixture of semi-solid hydrocarbons obtained from petroleum or heavy lubricating oil.

Yellow soft paraffin (Petrolatum; Petroleum jelly)

This a purified mixture of semisolid hydrocarbons obtained from petroleum. It may contain suitable stabilizers like, antioxidants e.g. α-tocopherol (Vitamin E), butylated hydroxy toluene (BHT) etc.

Melting range: 38^0C to 56^0C.

White soft paraffin (White petroleum jelly, White petrolatum)

This a purified mixture of semisolid hydrocarbons obtained from petroleum, and wholly or partially decolorized by percolating the yellow soft paraffin through freshly burned bone black or adsorptive clays.

Melting range: 38^0C to 56^0C.

Use: The white form is used when the medicament is colorless, white or a pastel shade. This base is used in

Dithranol ointment B.P.

Ammoniated Mercury and Coal tar ointment B.P.C.

Zinc ointment B.P.C.

(b) Hard paraffin (Paraffin)

This is a mixture of solid hydrocarbons obtained from petroleum.

It is colorless or white, odorless, translucent, wax-like substance. It solidifies between 50^0C and 57^0C and is used to stiffen ointment bases.

(c) Liquid paraffin (Liquid petrolatum; White mineral oil)

It is a mixture of liquid hydrocarbons obtained from petroleum. It is transparent, colorless, odorless, viscous liquid.

On long storage it may oxidize to produce peroxides and therefore, it may contain tocopherol or BHT as antioxidants.

It is used along with hard paraffin and soft paraffin to get a desired consistency of the ointment. Tubes for eye, rectal and nasal ointments have nozzles with narrow orifices through which it is difficult to expel very viscous ointments without the risk of bursting the tube. To facilitate the extrusion up to 25% of the base may be replaced by liquid paraffins.

Advantages of hydrocarbons bases:

(i) They are not absorbed by the skin. They remain on the surface as an occlusive layer that restricts the loss of moisture hence, keeps the skin soft.

(ii) They are sticky hence ensure prolonged contact between skin and medicament.

(iii) They are almost inert. They consist largely of saturated hydrocarbons, therefore, very few incompatibilities and little tendency of rancidity are encountered.

   (iv) They can withstand heat sterilization, hence, sterile ophthalmic ointments can be prepared with it.

   (v) They are readily available and cheap.

Disadvantages of hydrocarbon bases;

   (i) It may lead to water logging followed by maceration of the skin if applied for a prolonged period.

   (ii) It retains body heat, which may produce an uncomfortable feeling of warmth.

   (iii) They are immiscible with water; as a result, rubbing onto the surface and removal after treatment both are difficult.

   (iv) They are sticky, hence make application unpleasant and leads to contamination of clothes.

   (v) Water absorption capacity is very low, hence, these bases are poor in absorbing exudate from moist lesions.

Absorption Base

The term absorption base is used to denote the water absorbing or emulsifying property of these bases and not to describe their action on the skin.

These bases (sometimes called *emulsifiable ointment bases*) are generally anhydrous substances which have the property of absorbing (emulsifying) considerable quantity of water yet retaining its ointment-like consistency.

Preparations of this type do not contain water as a component of their basic formula but if water is incorporated a W/O emulsion is obtained.

Wool Fat (anhydrous lanolin)

It is the purified anhydrous fat like substance obtained from the wool of sheep.

- It is practically insoluble in water but can absorb water up to 50% of its own weight. Therefore, it is used in ointments the proportion of water or aqueous liquids to be incorporated in hydrocarbon base is too large.

- Due to its sticky nature it is not used alone but is used along with other bases in the preparation of a number of ointments.

e.g. Simple ointment B.P. contains 5% and the B.P. eye ointment base contains 10% wool fat.

Hydrous Wool Fat (Lanolin)

- It is a mixture of 70 % w/w wool fat and 30 % w/w purified water. It is a w/o emulsion. Aqueous liquids can be emulsified with it.

- It is used alone as an emollient.
- Example: - Hydrous Wool Fat Ointment B.P.C., Calamine Coal Tar Ointment.

Wool Alcohol

It is the emulsifying fraction of wool fat. Wool alcohol is obtained from wool fat by treating it with alkali and separating the fraction containing cholesterol and other alcohols. It contains not less than 30% of cholesterol.

Use:

- It is used as an emulsifying agent for the preparation of w/o emulsions and is used to absorb water in ointment bases.
- It is also used to improve the texture, stability and emollient properties of o/w emulsions.

Examples: - Wool alcohol ointment B.P. contains 6% wool alcohol and hard, liquid and soft paraffin.

Beeswax

It is purified wax, obtained from honey comb of bees.

It contains small amount of cholesterol. It is of two types: (a) yellow beeswax and (b) white beeswax. White bees wax is the bleached form of yellow bees wax. It may contain trace amount of bleaching agent and hence it is not used in ophthalmic ointments.

Use:

Beeswax is used as a stiffening agent in ointment preparations.

Examples: -Paraffin ointment B.P.C. contains beeswax.

Cholesterol

It is widely distributed in animal organisms. Wool fat is also used as a source of cholesterol.

Use: - It is used to increase the water absorbing power of an ointment base.

Example: - Hydrophilic petroleum U.S.P. contains:

Cholesterol	3% w/w
Stearyl alcohol	3% w/w
White beeswax	8% w/w
White soft paraffin	86% w/w

Advantages of absorption bases:
  (i)   They are less occlusive nevertheless, are good emollient.
  (ii)   They assist oil soluble medicaments to penetrate the skin.
  (iii) They are easier to spread.
  (iv)   They are compatible with majority of the medicaments.
  (v)   They are relatively heat stable.
  (vi)   The base may be used in their anhydrous form or in emulsified form.
  (vii) They can absorb a large quantity of water or aqueous substances.

Disadvantages: Inspite of their hydrophilic nature, absorption bases are difficult to wash.

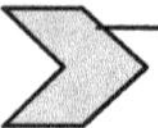 ## Water Miscible Bases

They are miscible with an excess of water. Ointments made from water-miscible bases are easily removed after use.

There are three official anhydrous water-miscible ointment bases: -

Example: -

Emulsifying ointment B.P. – contains anionic emulsifier.

Cetrimide emulsifying ointment B.P. – contains cationic emulsifier

Cetomacrogol emulsifying ointment B.P. – contains non-ionic emulsifier

Uses: they are used to prepare o/w creams and are easily removable ointment bases

e.g. Compound Benzoic Acid Ointment (Whitfield's Ointment) – used as antifungal ointment.

Advantages of water miscible bases:
  (i)   Readily miscible with the exudates from lesions.
  (ii)   Reduced interference with normal skin function.
  (iii) Good contact with the skin, because of their surfactant content.
  (iv)   High cosmetic acceptability, hence there is less likelihood of the patients discontinuing treatment.
  (v)   Easy removal from the hair.

Water Soluble Bases

Water soluble bases contain only the water-soluble ingredients and not the fats or other greasy substances, hence, they are known as grease-less bases.

Water soluble bases consists of water-soluble ingredients such as polyethylene glycol polymers (PEG) which are popularly known as "carbowaxes" and commercially known as "macrogols".

They are a range of compounds with the general formula:

$$CH_2OH.(CH_2OCH_2)_n CH_2OH$$

The PEGs are mixtures of polycondensation products of ethylene and water and they are described by numbers representing their average molecular weights. Like the paraffin hydrocarbons they vary in consistency from viscous liquids to waxy solids.

Example:

Macrogols 200, 300, 400   – viscous liquids

Macrogols 1500   – greasy semi-solids

Macrogols 1540, 3000, 4000, 6000   – waxy solids.

Different PEGs are mixed to get an ointment of desired consistency.

Advantages of PEGs as ointment base:

(a) They are water soluble; hence, very easily can be removed from the skin and readily miscible with tissue exudates.

(b) Helps in good absorption by the skin.

(c) Good solvent properties. Some water-soluble dermatological drugs, such as salicylic acid, sulfonamides, sulfur etc. are soluble in these bases.

(d) Non-greasy.

(e) They do not hydrolyze, rancidify or support microbial growth.

(f) Compatibility with many dermatological medicaments.

Disadvantages:

(a) Limited uptake of water. Macrogols dissolve when the proportion of water reaches about 5%.

(b) Reduction in activity of certain antibacterial agents, e.g. phenols, hydroxybenzoates and quaternary compounds.

(c) Solvent action on polyethylene and bake lite containers and closures.

Certain other substances which are used as water soluble ointment bases include tragacanth, gelatin, pectin, silica gel, sodium alginate, cellulose derivatives, etc.

Factors Governing Selection of an Ideal Ointment Base

1. *Dermatological factors*
2. *Pharmaceutical factors*

1. Dermatological factors

(a) *Absorption and Penetration*

'Penetration' means passage of the drug across the skin i.e. cutaneous penetration, and 'absorption' means passage of the drug into blood stream.

- Medicaments which are both soluble in oil and water are most readily absorbed though the skin.

- Animal and vegetable fats and oils normally penetrate the skin.

- Animals fats, e.g. lard and wool fat when combined with water, penetrates the skin.

- o/w emulsion bases release the medicament more readily than greasy bases or w/o emulsion bases.

(b) *Effect on the skin*

- Greasy bases interfere with normal skin functions i.e. heat radiation and sweating. They are irritant to the skin.

- o/w emulsion bases and other water miscible bases produce a cooling effect due to the evaporation of water.

(c) *Miscibility with skin secretion and serum*

Skin secretions are more readily miscible with emulsion bases than with greasy bases. Due to this the drug is more rapidly and completely released to the skin.

(d) *Compatibility with skin secretions*

The bases used should be compatible with skin secretions and should have pH about 5.5 because the average skin pH is around 5.5. Generally neutral ointment bases are preferred.

(e) *Non-irritant*

All bases should be highly pure and bases specially for eye ointments should be non-irritant and free from foreign particle.

(f) *Emollient properties*

Dryness and brittleness of the skin causes discomfort to the skin therefore, the bases should keep the skin moist. For this purpose, water and humectants such as glycerin, propylene glycol is used. Ointments should prevent rapid loss of moisture from the skin.

(g) *Ease of application and removal*

The ointment bases should be easily applicable as well as easily removable from the skin by simple washing with water. Stiff and sticky ointment bases require much force to spread on the skin and during rubbing newly formed tissues on the skin may be damaged.

2. Pharmaceutical factors

(a) *Stability*

Fats and oils obtained from animal and plant sources are prone to oxidation unless they are suitably preserved. This reaction is called *rancidification*. Lard, from animal origin, rancidify rapidly. Soft paraffin, simple ointment and paraffin ointment are inert and stable. Liquid paraffin is also stable but after prolonged storage it gets oxidized. Therefore, an antioxidant like *tocopherol* (Vit -E) may be incorporated. Other antioxidants those may be used are *butylated hydroxy toluene* (BHT) or *butylated hydroxy anisole* (BHA).

(b) *Solvent properties*

Most of the medicaments used in the preparation of ointments are insoluble in the ointment bases therefore, they are finely powdered and are distributed uniformly throughout the base.

(c) *Emulsifying properties*

Hydrocarbon bases absorbs very small amount of water.

Wool fat can take about 50% of water and when mixed with other fats can take up several times its own weight of aqueous solution.

Emulsifying ointment, cetrimide emulsifying ointment and cetomacrogol emulsifying ointment are capable of absorbing considerable amount of water, forming w/o creams.

(d) *Consistency*

The ointments produced should be of suitable consistency. They should neither be hard nor too soft. They should withstand climatic conditions. Thus, in summer they should not become too soft and in winter not too hard to be difficult to remove from the container and spread on the skin.

The consistency of an ointment base can be controlled by varying the ratio of hard and liquid paraffin.

Preparation of Ointments

A well-made ointment is –

(a) Uniform throughout i.e. it contains no lumps of separated high melting point ingredients of the base, there is no tendency for liquid constituents to separate and insoluble powders are evenly dispersed.

(b) Free from grittiness, i.e. insoluble powders are finely subdivided and large lumps of particles are absent. Methods of preparation must satisfy these criteria.

Two mixing techniques are frequently used in making ointments:

1. **Fusion**, in which ingredients are melted together and stirred to ensure homogeneity.

2. **Trituration**, in which finely-subdivided insoluble medicaments are evenly distributed by grinding with a small amount of the base or one of its ingredients followed by dilution with gradually increasing amounts of the base.

3. **Ointments prepared by Fusion method**:

   When an ointment base contains a number of solid ingredients such as white beeswax, cetyl alcohol, stearyl alcohol, stearic acid, hard paraffin, etc. as components of the base, it is required to melted them. The melting can be done in two methods:

   Method-I

   The components are melted in the decreasing order of their melting point i.e. the higher m.p. substance should be melted first, the substances with next melting point and so on. The medicament is added slowly in the melted ingredients and stirred thoroughly until the mass cools down and homogeneous product is formed.

   Advantages:

   This will avoid over-heating of substances having low melting point.

   Method-II

   All the components are taken in subdivided state and melted together.

   Advantages:

   The maximum temperature reached is lower than Method-I, and less time is required possibly due to the solvent action of the lower melting point substances on the rest of the ingredients.

Cautions:

   (i)   Melting time is shortened by grating waxy components (i.e. beeswax, wool alcohols, hard-paraffin, higher fatty alcohols and emulsifying waxes), by stirring during melting and by lowering the dish as far as possible into the water bath so that the maximum surface area is heated.

   (ii) The surface of some ingredients discolors due to oxidation e.g. wool fats and wool alcohols and this discolored layer should be removed before use.

   (iii) After melting, the ingredients should be stirred until the ointment is cool, taking care not to cause localized cooling, e.g. by using a cold spatula or stirrer, placing the dish on a cold surface (e.g. a plastic bench top) or transferring to a cold container before the ointment has fully set. If these precautions are ignored, hard lumps may separate.

   (iv) Vigorous-stirring, after the ointment has begun to thicken, causes excessive aeration and should be avoided.

(v) Because of their greasy nature, many constituents of ointment bases pickup dirt during storage, which can be seen after melting. This is removed from the melt by allowing it to sediment and decanting the supernatant, or by passage through muslin supported by a warm strainer. In both instances the clarified liquid is collected in another hot basin.

(vi) If the product is granular after cooling, due to separation of high m.p. constituents, it should be remelted, using the minimum of heat, and again stirred and cooled.

Example:

(i) Simple ointment B.P. contains

Wool fat	50 g
Hard paraffin	50 g
Cetostearyl alcohol	50 g
White soft paraffin	850 g

Type of preparation: Absorption ointment base

Procedure:

Hard paraffin and cetostearyl alcohol on water-bath. Wool fat and white soft paraffin are mixed and stirred until all the ingredients are melted.

If required decanted or strained and stirred until cold and packed in suitable container.

(ii) Paraffin ointment base

Type of preparation: Hydrocarbon ointment base

(iii) Wool alcohols ointment B.P.

Type of preparation: Absorption base

(iv) Emulsifying ointment B.P.

Type of preparation: Water-miscible ointment base.

(v) Macrogol ointment B.P.C

Type of preparation: Water soluble ointment base

Formula: Macrogol 4000

Liquid Macrogol 300

Method: Macrogol 4000 is melted and previously warmed liquid macrogol 300 is added. Stirred until cool.

2. Ointment Prepared by Trituration

This method is applicable in the base or a liquid present in small amount.

(i) Solids are finely powdered are passed through a sieve (# 250, # 180, #125).

(ii) The powder is taken on an ointment-slab and triturated with a small amount of the base. A steel spatula with long, broad blade is used. To this additional quantities of the base are incorporated and triturated until the medicament is mixed with the base.

(iii) Finally, liquid ingredients are incorporated. To avoid loss from splashing, a small volume of liquid is poured into a depression in the ointment and thoroughly incorporated before more is added in the same way. Splashing is more easily controlled in a mortar than on a tile.

Example:

(i) Whitfield ointment (Compound benzoic acid ointment B.P.C.)

Formula:	Benzoic acid, in fine powder	6 gm
	Salicylic acid, in fine powder	3 gm
	Emulsifying ointment	91 gm

Method: Benzoic acid and salicylic acid are sieved through No. 180 sieves. They are mixed on the tile with small amount of base and levigated until smooth and diluted gradually.

3. Ointment Preparation by Chemical Reaction

Chemical reactions were involved in the preparation of several famous ointments of the past, e.g. Strong Mercuric Nitrate Ointment, 1959 B.P.C.

(a) Ointment containing free iodine

Iodine is only slightly soluble in most fats and oils but readily soluble.

Iodine is readily soluble in concentrated solution of potassium iodide due to the formation of molecular complexes $KI.I_2$, $KI.2I_2$, $KI.3I_2$ etc.

These solutions may be incorporated in absorption-type ointment bases.

e.g. *Strong Iodine Ointment B.Vet.C* (British Veterinary Pharmacopoeia) is used to treat ringworm in cattle. It contains free iodine. At one time this type of ointments was used as counter-irritants in the treatment of human rheumatic diseases but they were not popular because:

(i) They stain the skin a deep red color.

(ii) Due to improper storage, the water dries up and the iodine crystals irritate the skin, hence glycerol was used some times to dissolve the iodine-potassium iodide complex instead of water.

Example: Strong Iodine Ointment B. 7% Vet.C.

Iodine	7% w/v
Woolfat	50% w/v
Yellow soft paraffin	35% w/v
Potassium iodide	5% w/v
Water	q.s

Procedure:

(i)   KI is dissolved in water. I_2 is dissolved in it.

(ii) Wool fat and yellow soft paraffin are melted together over water bath. Melted mass is cooled to about 40^0C.

(iii) I_2 solution is added to the melted mass in small quantities at a time with continuous stirring until a uniform mass is obtained.

(iv) It is cooled to room temperature and packed.

Use: - Ringworm in cattle.

(b) Ointment containing combined iodine

Fixed oils and many vegetable and animal fats absorb iodine which combines with the double bonds of the unsaturated constituents, e.g.

$$CH_3.(CH_2)_2.CH = CH.(CH_2)_7.COOH + I_2 \rightarrow CH_3.(CH_2)_2.CHI\ CHI.(CH_2)_7.COOH$$

Oleic acid   di-iodostearic acid

Example: Non-staining Iodine Ointment B.P.C. 1968   Iodine
Arachis Oil
Yellow Soft Paraffin

Method:

(a) Iodine is finely powdered in a glass mortar and required amount is added to the oil in a glass-stoppered conical flask and stirred well.

(b) The oil is heated at 50^0C in a water-bath and stirred continually. Heating is continued until the brown color is changed to greenish-black; this may take several hours.

(c) From 0.1g of the preparation the amount of iodine is determined by B.P.C. method and the amount of soft paraffin base is calculated to give the product the required strength.

(d) Soft paraffin is warmed to 40^0C. The iodized oil is added and mixed well. No more heat is applied because this causes deposition of a resinous substance.

(e) The preparation is packed in a warm, wide-mouthed, amber color, glass bottle. It is allowed to cool without further stirring.

4. Preparation of Ointments by Emulsification

An emulsion system contains an oil phase, an aqueous phase and an emulsifying agent.

For o/w emulsion systems the following emulsifying agents are used:

(i)   water soluble soap

(ii) cetyl alcohol

(iii) glyceryl monostearate

(iv) combination of emulsifiers: triethanolamine stearate + cetyl alcohol

(v) non-ionic emulsifiers: glyceryl monostearate, glyceryl monooleate, propylene glycol stearate

For w/o emulsion creams the following emulsifiers are used:

(i) polyvalent ions e.g. *magnesium, calcium and aluminium* are used.

(ii) combination of emulsifiers: *beeswax + divalent calcium ion*

The viscosity of this type of creams prevent coalescence of the emulsified phases and helps in stabilizing the emulsion.

Example:

Cold cream

Procedure:

(i) Water immiscible components e.g. oils, fats, waxes are melted together over water bath (70^0C).

(ii) Aqueous solution of all heat stable, water soluble components are heated (70^0C).

(iii) Aqueous solution is slowly added to the melted bases with continuous stirring until the product cools down and a semi-solid mass is obtained.

N.B. The aqueous phase is heated otherwise high melting point fats and waxes will immediately solidify on addition of cold aqueous solution.

Stability of Ointments

The ointments should remain stable from the time of preparation to the time when the whole of it is consumed by the user.

(i) To stop microbial growth, preservatives are added for ointment which includes: p-hydroxy benzoates, phenol, benzoic acid, sorbic acid, methyl paraben, propyl paraben, quaternary ammonium compounds, mercury compounds etc.

(ii) The preservatives should not react with any of the component of the formulation. Plastic containers may absorb the preservative and thereby decreasing the concentration of preservative available for killing the bacteria.

(iii) Some ingredients like wool fat and wool alcohols are susceptible to oxidation. Therefore, a suitable antioxidant may be incorporated to protect the active ingredients from oxidation.

(iv) Incompatible drugs, emulsifying agents and preservatives must be avoided. The drugs which are likely to hydrolyze must be dispensed in an anhydrous base.

(v) Humectants such as, glycerin, propylene glycol and sorbitol may be added to prevent the loss of moisture from the preparation.

(vi) Ointment must be stored at an optimum temperature otherwise separation of phases may take place in the emulsified products which may be very difficult to remix to get a uniform product.

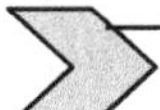

Practical Based on Ointments

1. AIM- To prepare iodine ointment, non-staining (20g)

Ingredients	Qty prescribed (1000g)	Qty used (20g)
Iodine	50g	1g
Arachis oil	150.0ml	3ml
Yellow soft paraffin q.s.	1000g	20g

Theory- Ointments are semisolid dosage forms containing drug in soluble or dispersed form. They are meant for application to the skin. Iodine ointment contains iodine as an analgesic and antiseptic component; arachis oil as an unsaturated fatty acid ($C_{20}H_{32}O_2$) and yellow soft paraffin as a hydrocarbon ointment base which is greasy, smooth and occlusive.

$$CH_3\text{-}(CH_2)_2\text{-}CH=CH\text{-}(CH_2)_2\text{-}CH=CH\text{-}(CH_2)_2\text{-}CH=CH\text{-}(CH_2)_2\text{-}CH=Ch\text{-}(CH_2)_2\text{-}Ch_3 + I_2 \longrightarrow$$

$$CH_3\text{-}(CH_2)_2\text{-}CH=CH\text{-}(CH_2)_2\text{-}CH=CH\text{-}(CH_2)_2\text{-}CH=CH\text{-}(CH_2)_2\text{-}CH=CH\text{-}(CH_2)_2\text{-}CH_3$$

Arachis oil is an unsaturated fatty acid which pairs up with the molecular iodine resulting in formation of polyiodoarachistonic acid; as a result, no free iodine is available. Thus, no stain is produced when such ointment is used due to absence of free iodine.

Procedure: Shake iodine with arachis oil at room temperature until it dissolves completely. Maintain the solution at 50°C with occasional stirring until the brown color disappears. Add sufficient quantity of yellow soft paraffin previously heated to 40°C to produce the final weight.

Uses: Topical Antiseptic

Storage: Keep in cool and dry place away from sunlight

Close the bottle tightly after use

Precautions: FOR EXTERNAL USE ONLY

2. AIM- To Prepare methyl salicylate and iodine ointment (20 g)

Ingredients used	Qty prescribed (1000 g)	Qty used (20 g)
Methyl Salicylate	50 ml	1 ml
Non-staining iodine Ointment q.s.	1000 g	20 g

Theory: Methyl salicylate is also known as oil of wintergreen, neelgiri ka tel, or betula oil & methyl-2-hydroxy benzoate. It is widely used in a number of formulations as a rubefacient and analgesic to treat deep seated pain. Iodine is also used for its analgesic effect. Paraffin is used as a base which provides a greasy, smooth and occlusive cover over the applied area. This formulation is used for treatment of deep-seated pain or as a muscle relaxant. Methyl salicylate is known to soften the plastic containers in which it is stored, so this formulation should be stored only in glass containers.

Procedure: Melt non-staining iodine ointment at lower temperature and add methyl salicylate. Mix and cool.

Uses: Topical Analgesic and antiseptic.

Precautions: FOR EXTERNAL USE ONLY

3. AIM- To prepare White Ointment (20 g)

Ingredients used	Qty prescribed (1000 g)	Qty used (20 g)
White Wax	50 g	1 g
Petrolatum	950 g	19 g

Procedure: Melt white wax in china dish and add petrolatum in it and warm until liquefaction. Discontinue heating and continue stirring so as to congeal the mass.

Uses: Emollient, as vehicle for other ointments.

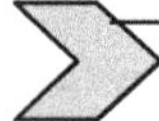 **Gels**

Pharmaceutical gels are often simple phase, transparent semi-solid systems that are being increasingly used as pharmaceutical topical formulations. The liquid phase of the gel may be retained within a three-dimensional polymer matrix. Drugs can be suspended in the matrix or dissolved in the liquid phase.

Advantages of gels

✓ Stable over long periods of time

✓ Good appearance

✓ Suitable vehicles for applying medicaments to skin and mucous membranes giving high rates of release of the medicament and rapid absorption.

Examples: Anaesthetic gels, Coal tar gels for use in treatment of psoriasis or eczema, Lubricant gels, Spermicidal gels.

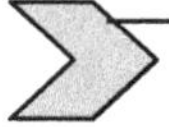 **Pastes**

(i) Pastes generally contains a large amount (50%) of finely powdered solids. So they are often stiffer than ointments.

(ii) When applied to the skin, pastes adhere well, forming a thick coating protects and soothes inflamed and raw surfaces and minimizes the damage done by scratching in itchy conditions such as chronic eczema. it is comparatively easy to confine pastes to the diseased areas whereas ointments, which are usually less viscous, tend to spread on to healthy skin, and this may result in sensitivity reactions if the preparations contain a powerful medicament such as *dithranol.*

(iii) Because of the powder contents pastes are porous; hence, perspiration can escape. Since the powders absorbs exudate, pastes with hydrocarbon base are less macerating than ointments with a similar base.

(iv) They are less greasy than ointments but since their efficacy depends on maintaining a thick surface layer they are far from attractive cosmetically.

(v) Most of the pastes are unsuitable for treating scalp conditions because they are difficult to remove from the hair.

Bases of Pastes

1. Hydrocarbon base:

Soft paraffin and liquid paraffin are commonly used bases for the preparation of paste.

	Name of the preparation	Active ingredients	Base	Use
1.	Compound Zinc Paste B.P.	Zinc oxide	Soft paraffin	Eczema,
2.	Compound Zinc & Salicylic acid Paste B.P. (Lassar's Paste)	Zinc oxide & Salicylic acid	Soft paraffin	psoriasis. Eczema,
3.	Coal tar paste	Coal tar	Soft paraffin	psoriasis.
4.	Dithranol paste compound	Dithranol	Soft paraffin	Eczema
5.	Aluminium paste B.P.C. (Baltimore Paste)	Aluminium oxide	Liquid paraffin	Ring worm or psoriasis Protectant

2. Water miscible base:

Name of the preparation	Base	Use
1. Resorcinol & sulfur Paste B.P.C. 2. Zinc & Coal tar Paste 3. Magnesium sulfate paste B.P.C. (Morison's paste) 4. Titanium dioxide paste B.P.C.	Emulsifying ointment Emulsifying wax Magnesium sulfate - 45% Phenol in glycerol Suspension of TiO_2, ZnO, light kaolin and red Fe_2O_3 in glycerol + water.	Dandruff, and are easily removable from the hair. Eczema Used to treat boils, because of their powerful osmotic effect of the salt and the glycerol. Absorbs exudates from weeping skin conditions.

3. Water soluble bases

Water soluble bases are prepared from mixtures of high and low molecular weight polyethylene glycols (or macrogols).

Name of the preparation	Base	Use
1. Water soluble dental pastes 2. Triamcinolone Dental paste B.P.C.	Neomycin sulfate Triamcinolone acetonide in an adhesive paste (NaCMC, pectin, + gelatin)	Sterilizing infected root canal Anti-inflammatory

Methods of Preparation

Like ointment, pastes are prepared by trituration and fusion methods. Trituration method is used when the base is liquid or semisolid.

Fusion method is used when the base is semisolid and/or solid in nature.

Preparation 1.

Name: **Compound Zinc Paste**

Formula	Zinc oxide, finely sifted	25 g
	Starch, finely sifted	25 g
	White soft paraffin	50 g

Type of preparation: Paste with semi-solid base prepared by fusion and trituration.

Procedure:

(a) Zinc oxide and starch powder are passed through No. 180 sieve.

(b) Soft paraffin is melted on a water bath.

(c) The required amount of powder is taken in a warm mortar, triturated with little melted base until it becomes smooth. Gradually, rest of the base is added and mixed until cold.

Preparation 2.

Name: **Zinc and Coal-tar Paste B.P.C.**

Formula: Zinc oxide, finely sifted   60 g

     Coal tar   60 g

     Emulsifying wax   50 g

     Starch   380 g

     Yellow soft paraffin   450 g

Type of preparation: Paste with semi-solid base prepared by fusion.

Procedure:

Method-I

(a) Emulsifying wax is melted in a tared dish (70^0C).

(b) The coal tar is weighed in the dish. Stirred to mix.

   Soft paraffin is melted in a separate dish (70^0C) and about half is added to the tar-wax mixture; stirred well. Remainder is added; stirred again until homogeneous.

   Allowed to cool at about (30^0C) and zinc oxide (previously passed through 180 mesh) and starch, in small amount with constant stirring. Stirred until cold.

Method-II

Wax and paraffin melted together, mixed well and stirred until just setting. Powders are mixed on a slightly warm tile and the tar is incorporated. This method eliminates the risk of overheating.

practical Based on Pastes

1. AIM- To prepare Unnan's Paste

Theory: The paste consists of gelatin as a base. Gelatin solution is formed on heating and turns to gel form on cooling down providing stiffness to the base. Glycerin is used as a preservative to prevent pure faction of gelatin, it also acts as non-volatile hygroscopic emollient. Zinc oxide acts as astringent and skin protective. The paste is hard in consistency and is should be melted before use. It is applied using a stiff brush.

Ingredients	Quantity prescribed	Quantity used
Zinc Oxide (Sifted)	15 g	4.8 g
Gelatin	15 g	4.8 g
Glycerin	35 ml	11.2 ml
Purified water	35 ml	11.2 ml

Procedure:

- Heat purified water in a china dish on a water bath and sprinkle gelatin over it with continuous stirring to completely mix gelatin.
- Heat glycerin in another china dish and add hot glycerin to the gelatin solution slowly to avoid air entrapment.
- Weigh the content of dish and add additional water if necessary to make up the content.
- Sift zinc oxide through sieve no. 60 and incorporate to the molten base in small portions.
- Continue the stirring without aeration. Pour the contents on a shallow tray and allow a film to be formed which could be cut into small pieces for storage.

Storage: Cut the pieces into ¼ in square pieces and store in a wide mouth jar.

Direction for use: Melt appropriate number of pieces and apply on affected area using a brush and cover it with a gauge bandage.

Precautions: For external use only

Uses: Mild astringent, Protective

2. **To prepare Lassar's Paste**

Ingredients	Quantity prescribed	Quantity used
Zinc Oxide (Sifted)	24 g	5.3 g
Salicylic Acid (Sifted)	2 g	0.44 g
Starch (Sifted)	24 g	5.3 g
White Soft Paraffin	50 g	11 g

Theory: It is a combination paste consisting of zinc oxide and salicylic acid. Salicylic acid acts as antifungal and zinc oxide acts as astringent, soothing agent and topical protective. Starch acts as adsorbent and gives stiffness to the paste.

Zinc oxide, salicylic acid and starch are insoluble in white soft paraffin. Therefore, lassar's paste is prepared by combining fusion and trituration method.

Procedure: Melt white soft paraffin, in a china dish over a water bath. Sift zinc oxide, salicylic acid and starch through sieve no. 60 to get a fine powder and mix them uniformly. Add the sifted mixture to the melted white soft paraffin and mix them properly until it forms a homogeneous paste.

Direction: Apply paste to the affected part three to four times a day.

Precaution: For external use only.

Uses: Topical antifungal, protective, astringent.

3. AIM- To prepare Sulfanilamide Paste

Ingredients	Qty prescribed
Sulfanilamide	7.5 g
Pectin	4.5 g
Glycerin	12.0 g
Normal Saline Solution q.s.	50.0 g

Procedure: Triturate sulfanilamide, pectin and glycerin. In a separate beaker heat normal saline to its boiling and add with stirring in the triturated mixture until it takes a consistency of a thick paste.

Direction: Apply paste on the affected area 2-3 times a day

Uses: Topical antiseptic

FOR EXTERNAL USE ONLY

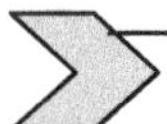

Creams

These are semi-solid emulsions for external use.

Classification of creams:

✓ Aqueous cream (o/w type)

✓ Oily cream (w/o type)

They do not stain the skin.

Aqueous creams: The emulsion is o/w type. These creams are relatively non-greasy.

(a) Creams containing *anionic emulsifying agent*:

Emulsifiers: Anionic emulsifiers e.g. Emulsifying ointment

(b) Creams containing *cationic emulsifying agent*:

Emulsifiers: Cationic emulsifiers e.g. Cetyl trimethyl ammonium bromide (Cetrimide)

(c) Creams containing *nonionic emulsifying agent*:

Emulsifiers: Monostearin, sorbitan esters (polysorbates), fatty alcohols (like stearyl alcohol)

Procedure:

(i) Oil phase containing oils, waxes are melted together at 70^0C.

(ii) Aqueous phase containing water-soluble ingredients, emulsifying agents are dissolved in water and temperature is raised to 70^0C on a water bath.

(iii) Aqueous phase is mixed to oil phase. Constantly stirred until cooled.

Oily creams: The emulsion is w/o type. These creams are greasy in nature.

(a) *Sterol creams:* Emulsifiers: – Wool fat, wool alcohol.

(b) *Soap creams*: Emulsifiers: – Triethanol amine soap, Borax soap.

Procedure:

(i) Oil phase containing oils, waxes and emulsifying agent are melted together at 70⁰C.

(ii) Aqueous phase containing water-soluble ingredients are dissolved in water and temperature is raised to 70⁰C on a water bath.

(iii) Aqueous phase is mixed to oil phase. Constantly stirred until cooled.

Containers: Wide mouthed, air-tight jars.

Label: FOR EXTERNAL USE ONLY,   *"Store in a cool place"*

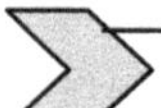

Practicals Based on Creams

1. AIM- To prepare Cold Cream (10ml)

Ingredients	Qty prescribed
White Bees Wax	10 g
Liquid Paraffin	30 g
Borax	0.5 g
Rose Oil	0.1 ml
Water	10 ml

Theory: It is water in oil type emulsion which provides a cooling effect on skin on application due to slow evaporation of water. It is prepared by saponification reaction between beeswax (fatty acid) and borax (alkali) which forms a soap in situ which acts as emulsifying agent. Liquid paraffin is used as emollient and rose oil is used as perfume.

Procedure: Grate small pieces of beeswax and weigh the required quantity in a china dish along with liquid paraffin. Dissolve borax in water in beaker and heat up to 70 °C. When both phases are at same temperature, gradually add borax solution to the melt of beeswax with constant stirring.

Direction: Apply to skin as per requirement

Storage: Keep in cool and dry place, Do not freeze

Auxiliary Label: FOR EXTERNAL USE ONLY

Uses: As emollient, treatment of dry skin

2. AIM- To prepare Vanishing Cream

Ingredients	Qty prescribed
Stearic Acid	25.0 g
Potassium Hydroxide	0.8 g
Glycerin	10.0 ml
Methyl Paraben	0.2 g
Water	64.0 ml

Theory: It is oil in water type emulsion which when applied to skin vanishes and leaves an almost invisible layer on it. The layer which is left behind acts as a base or foundation for facial make up, hence they are also known as foundation creams. The main ingredients are stearic acid, alkali and water. stearic acid gives it the shining appearance. Soap is prepared *in situ* by reaction of stearic acid and alkali which emulsifies the oil phase in water.

Procedure: Melt stearic acid in a china dish and heat on a water bath to 70°C. Dissolve potassium hydroxide and methyl paraben in water and add glycerin to it and take its temperature to 70°C. Add aqueous phase to the melted stearic acid with continuous stirring, remove the china dish from and heat and keep on stirring continuously until it becomes cool and a homogenous cream is obtained.

Direction: Apply to skin as per requirement

Storage: Keep in cool and dry place

Auxiliary Label: FOR EXTERNAL USE ONLY

Uses: As a foundation, for holding makeup for longer period of time.

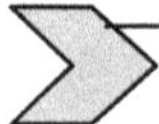 **Unit 6**

Miscellaneous Topics

List of Some Useful Books and Reference Materials

(Latest Editions)

- ❖ Indian Pharmacopoeia and National Formularies (N.F.I., RN.F.), Govt. of India Publication
- ❖ British Pharmacopoeia.
- ❖ The United States Pharmacopeia - National Formulary by United States Pharmacopeial Convention
- ❖ Alfonso R. Gennaro Remington. The Science and Practice of Pharmacy, Lippincott Williams, New Delhi
- ❖ Martindale- The Extra Pharmacopoeia
- ❖ Ansel's Pharmaceutical Dosage Forms and Drug Delivery Systems by Loyd Allen, Lippincott Williams and Walkins, New Delhi
- ❖ Aulton's Pharmaceutics by Michael E. Aulton (Editor); Kevin M. G. Taylor (Editor) Pharmaceutics, The Science & Dosage Form Design, Churchill Livingstone, Edinburgh
- ❖ Pharmaceutical Compounding and Dispensing by John Marriott; Dawn Belcher; Keith A. Wilson; Christopher A. Langley
- ❖ Pharmaceutical Calculations by Howard C. Ansel; Shelly J. Stockton
- ❖ Cooper and Gunn's Dispensing for Pharmaceutical Students by Carter SJ, CBS publishers, New Delhi
- ❖ Carter S.J., Cooper and Gunn's. Tutorial Pharmacy, CBS Publications, New Delhi
- ❖ Shayne Cox Gad-Pharmaceutical Manufacturing Handbook
- ❖ History of Pharmacy in India by Dr. Harikishan Singh
- ❖ Bentleys' Text book of Pharmaceutics, 8th Edition, editor E.A. Rawlins, published by Elsevier Int.
- ❖ The Theory and Practice of Industrial Pharmacy. Leon Lachman, Herbert Lieberman and Joseph Kanig, Editors, Lea and Febiger, Philadelphia. Latest edition Verghese Publishing House.

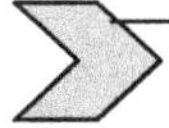 **Glossary**

Application A liquid or semi-liquid preparation intended for application to the skin.

Bougie – nasal A solid dosage form intended for insertion into the nostril.

Bougie – urethral A solid dosage form intended for insertion into the urethra.

Cachet An oral preparation consisting of dry powder enclosed in a shell of rice paper.

Capsule An oral preparation consisting of a medicament enclosed in a shell, usually of gelatin basis. Soft gelatin capsules are used to enclose liquids and hard capsules to enclose solids.

Cream A semi-solid emulsion intended for application to the skin. The emulsion may be an oil-in-water emulsion (aqueous creams) or water-in-oil type (oily creams).

Douche A liquid preparation intended for introduction into the vagina.

Douche – nasal A liquid preparation intended for introduction into the nostril.

Draught A liquid oral preparation of fairly small volume and usually consisting of one dose.

Drops A liquid preparation in which the quantity to be used at any one time is so small that it is measured as a number of drops, e.g. in a small pipette. Drops may comprise an oral preparation, usually paediatric, or may be intended for introduction into the nose, ear or eye, where the title of the product is amended accordingly.

Dusting powder A preparation consisting of one or more substances in fine powder intended for the application to intact skin.

Elixir An aromatic liquid preparation including a high proportion of alcohol, glycerine, propylene glycol or other solvent, and intended for the oral administration of potent or nauseous medicaments, in a small dose volume.

Emulsion As a preparation, this term is generally restricted to an oil-in water preparation intended for internal use.

Enema An aqueous or oily solution or suspension intended for rectal administration.

Gargle An aqueous solution, usually in concentrated form, intended for the treatment of the membranous lining of the throat.

Granules A dry preparation in which each granule consists of a mixture of the ingredients in the correct proportions.

Inhalation A preparation in which the active principle is drawn into the respiratory tract by inhalation. The active principle may be vapour when it is obtained from a liquid preparation by volatilisation, or it may be a solid when a special appliance, often an aerosol, is needed.

Injection A preparation intended for parenteral administration which may consist of an aqueous or non-aqueous solution or suspension.

Irrigation A solution intended for introduction into body cavities or deep wounds which includes nasal and vaginal douches.

Levigation This is the term applied to the incorporation into the base of insoluble coarse powders. It is often termed 'wet grinding'. It is the process where the powder is rubbed down with either the molten base or semi-solid base. A considerable shearing force is applied to avoid a gritty product.

Linctus A viscous liquid preparation, usually containing sucrose, which is administered in small dose volumes and which should be sipped and swallowed slowly without the addition of water.

Liniment A liquid or semi-liquid intended for application to intact skin, usually with considerable friction produced by massaging with the hand.

Lotion A liquid preparation intended for application to the skin without friction. Eye lotions are lotions intended for application to the eye.

Lozenge A solid oral preparation consisting of medicaments incorporated in a flavoured base and intended to dissolve or disintegrate slowly in the mouth.

Mixture Liquid oral preparation consisting of one or more medicaments dissolved, suspended or diffused in an aqueous vehicle.

Mouthwash An aqueous solution, often in concentrated form, intended for local treatment of the membranous lining of the mouth and gums.

Ointment A semi-solid preparation consisting of one or more medicaments dissolved or dispersed in a suitable base and intended for application to the skin.

Paint A liquid preparation intended for application to the skin or mucous membranes.

Pastille A solid oral preparation consisting of one or medicaments in an inert base and intended to dissolve slowly in the mouth.

Pessary A solid dosage form intended for insertion into the vagina for local treatment.

Pill A solid oral dose form consisting of one or more medicaments incorporated in a spherical or ovoid mass.

Poultice A thick pasty preparation intended for application to the skin whilst hot.

Powder A preparation consisting of one or more components in fine powder. It may be in bulk form or individually wrapped quantities and is intended for oral administration.

Suppository A solid dosage form intended for insertion into the rectum for local or systemic treatment.

Syrup A liquid preparation containing a high proportion of sucrose or other sweetening agent.

Tablet A solid oral dosage form where one or more medicaments are compressed and moulded into shape.

Appendices

Some Common Abbreviations

Abbreviation	Latin form	Meaning
aa.	ana	of each
a.c.	ante cibum	before food
ad/add	addendus	to be added (up to)
ad lib	ad libitum	as much as desired
alt	alternus	alternate
alt die	alterno die	every other day
amp	ampulla	ampoule
applic	applicetur	let it be applied
aq	aqua	water
aq ad	aquam ad	water up to
aur/aurist	auristillae	ear drops
bd/bid	bis in die	twice a day
c	cum	with
cap	capsula	capsule
cc	cum cibus	with food
co/comp	compositus	compound
collut	collutorium	mouthwash
conc	concentratus	concentrated
corp	corpori	to the body
crem	cremor	cream
d	dies	a day

Nominal pH values of some body fluids and sites

Site	Nominal pH
Aqueous humour	7.21
Blood	7.40
Cerebrospinal fluid	7.35
Duodenum	7.35
Ileum	8.00
Colon	5.5-7.0
Tear (Lacrimal fluid)	7.4
saliva	6.4
Semen	7.2
Stomach	1-3
Urine	5.6-5.8
Vaginal secretion (Premenopause)	4.5
Vaginal secretion (Postmenopause)	7.0

pK$_a$ values of some typical acidic and basic drugs

(Source: Martindale: The Extra Pharmacopoeia)

Acidic Drugs	pK$_a$	Basic Drugs	pK$_a$
Acetylsalicylic acid	3.5	Amphetamine	9.8
Barbital	7.9	Atropine	9.7
Phenobarbital	7.4	Quinine	4.2, 8.8
Penicillin G	2.8	Codeine	7.9
Phenytoin	8.3	Morphine	7.9
Theophylline	8.6	Procaine	9.0
Tolbutamide	5.3	Verapamil	8.8

Log P Values of Some Typical Drugs

The logarithm of partition coefficient (P) is known as *log P*. Log P is a measure of lipophilicity and is used widely, since many pharmaceutical and biological events depend on lipophilic characteristics. Often, the log P of a compound is quoted. The lists the log P values of some representative compounds. For a given drug:

If log $P = 0$, there is equal drug distribution in both phases.

If log $P > 0$, the drug is lipid soluble.

If log $P < 0$, the drug is water soluble.

Drug	LogP
Acetylsalicylic acid	1.19
Amiodarone	6.7
Benzocaine	1.89
Bromocriptine	6.6
Bupivacaine	3.4
Caffeine	0.01
Chlorpromazine	5.3
Cortisone	1.47
Desipramine	4.0
Glutethimide	1.9
Haloperidol	1.53
Hydrocortisone	4.3
Indomethacin	3.1
Lidocaine	2.26
Methadone	3.9
Misoprostol	2.9
Ondansetron	3.2

Contd...

Drug	LogP
Pergolide	3.8
Phenytoin	2.5
Physostigmine	2.2
Prednisone	1.46
Sulfadimethoxine	1.56
Sulfadiazine	0.12
Sulfathiazole	0.35
Tetracaine	3.56
Thiopentone	2.8
Xamoterol	0.5
Zimelidine	2.7